Of Bears
& Weight Loss

HOW TO MANAGE
TRIGGERS, LOSE WEIGHT,
AND ENJOY GETTING FIT

Of Bears & Weight Loss

Dr. Brian King

PSYCHOLOGIST AND COMEDIAN

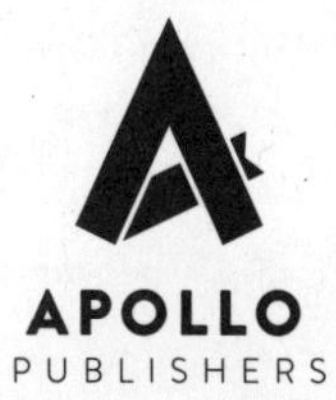

APOLLO
PUBLISHERS

Of Bears and Weight Loss:

How to Manage Triggers, Lose Weight, and Enjoy Getting Fit

 All inquiries should be sent by email to Apollo Publishers at info@apollopublishers.com. Apollo Publishers books may be purchased for educational, business, or sales promotional use. Special editions may be made available upon request. For details, contact Apollo Publishers at info@apollopublishers.com.

Visit our website at www.apollopublishers.com.

Published in compliance with California's Proposition 65.

Library of Congress Control Number: 2022941618

Print ISBN: 978-1-954641-22-8

Ebook ISBN: 978-1-954641-23-5

Printed in the United States of America.

For Sarah and Alyssa, thank you for giving me the motivation I needed and for helping me along the way.

Contents

CHAPTER 4

CHAPTER 5

CHAPTER 6

CHAPTER 7

Bonjour de Montréal

I hope that by writing this I don't accidentally encourage a ton of new people to relocate to Montreal, Quebec. Massive influxes of new citizens can change the feel of a city. I've seen it happen in others that I've lived in and loved. Not that I had anything to do with it, but Austin, Texas, became unrecognizable soon after I finished college there. New Orleans, San Francisco, and Portland all saw population booms while I was living within each of their borders, and I watched the cultures of all three change right in front of me. I would hate to have this happen to my beautiful Montreal and that is certainly not my intention. But as I sit looking out my window onto the historic plaza that doubles as my front yard and attempt to gather my thoughts and notes for this book, all I keep returning to is how great it is to be here.

I first came to Montreal after my last year of college. I was working as a counselor at a summer camp about two hours upstate from New York City. It was the kind of job that college students take more for the experiences than the money. As I traveled all the way to New York from my college in Texas for camp counselor wages, clearly I was in it for those experiences.

About every two weeks the campers would go home and the staff members would have a few days off to do as we pleased. Some chose to stay at the camp, enjoying quiet time in nature, but most of us headed down to New York City to do all the things that people do there. One break, however, I decided to point my car north. Another counselor was a student at McGill University in Montreal, and after telling him I had never been there, he offered me a chance to stay at his apartment, which otherwise was going to be empty all summer. My brother, Jon, who also worked at the camp that year, decided to join me, as did two of our friends from New York, and we spent a long weekend exploring this amazing French-speaking city to the north.

I felt as if we had flown across the Atlantic, when all it really took was a few hours in the car. Even though we didn't speak French, my friends and I managed to get by, finding ourselves barhopping, sightseeing, and perpetually smiling for the entire weekend.

I absolutely loved it and always expressed a desire to return. However, life got in the way, as it tends to do. I finished college in Austin, graduate school in New Orleans and Ohio, and started working in Pennsylvania before moving to California, Oregon, and back to California. A full twenty years passed before I made it back to Montreal, driving over after a tour of the New England states. A little bit older and slightly more sober, I was reminded of how beautiful the city is. I spent most of my time in Old Montreal, eating and drinking Bloody Caesars,[1] and promised myself not to let another twenty years pass before my next visit.

Two years later, I made good on that promise. This time with

1 I was writing a book! It was research, I assure you.

my new girlfriend, Sarah, along for the ride. We stayed for a month, and with the extra time we discovered Montreal's festival season. Our favorites were the MURAL Festival, which annually transforms buildings around town into works of art; the Montreal Jazz Festival, which offers amazing concerts every night for free; the Cirque Festival, which we stumbled onto after witnessing a circus performer flash mob; and of course the Just for Laughs Comedy Festival. In between, we explored city parks and museums and had so much fun that by the time we left one of us was pregnant. I'll let you guess which one.

We came back the following year, this time with our barely three-month-old daughter, Alyssa, and spent about two months in a neighborhood called Le Plateau-Mont-Royal. For the few years before that summer, I had been thinking of putting down some roots somewhere; but I hadn't yet found a place that felt right. Now that I had a family, establishing roots was on my mind more than ever. I had never before considered buying a home outside of my country of birth (especially not my first home), but that stay reaffirmed our love for a city full of art and culture, and for each other. We wanted to own a piece of it and be a part of it. Some very effective signs around the neighborhood and curiosity led us to pop into a local real estate office on a goof. I can only imagine how we appeared when we walked in, an English-speaking American couple pushing a stroller, but the agent took the time to show us some properties anyway, and he guided us through the French-Canadian real estate process. By the time we left town, we owned a small condo in a wonderful neighborhood. It would be years before we had an opportunity to use it, which is ironic as our initial intent was to drop some roots, but that is where I am now.

Last month, after spending a few years away from Montreal, my family drove halfway across the United States and returned to the city and condo we'd fallen in love with, for the purpose of my writing this book on weight management. And yes, it is great to be here—although after having indulged in a few poutines,[2] I am starting to question that decision.

2 I'll share more about these later, but if you don't know poutine, it is a Montreal specialty consisting of french fries topped with cheese curds and covered in gravy.

1

Three Books

Who am I, anyway? You can probably tell from what I've written so far that I've moved around a lot. And in more than one way. I've changed careers almost as often as I've changed zip codes. One time while onstage, I asked a man in the audience what he did for a living, and he told me he was a limousine driver. So I asked him how he got into that, and he said, "Believe it or not, I used to drive a taxi!" Do you need the phrase "believe it or not" in this situation? I think that's a pretty obvious career path. I would have also accepted bus driver. Save the phrase "believe it or not" for when you have something truly unbelievable to tell me, like "Believe it or not, I used to be a wet nurse!" Believe it or not, I am just a typical psychologist turned comedian turned public speaker turned author turned wet nurse.[3] That actually sounds like a ridiculous career path when I lay it all out in a single sentence,

3 Someday, hopefully. A boy can dream. If so, would this qualify as a wet dream?

and it would even if I cut out the one that isn't true; but living it felt a lot more organic.

I was the first person on both sides of my family to go to college. My parents had suggested I go to trade school or follow in the family tradition and join the military, but being the rebellious kid I was, I decided to enroll at the University of Texas at Austin. When I started, I had no idea what kind of career I wanted to pursue, and that may help explain my path a bit. I wanted to be an artist, writer, and comedian, but I knew those roads would be difficult to follow and didn't required advance education, so I took classes in whatever interesting subjects fit my schedule until it was time to pick a major. I settled on psychology because I had accumulated more credits toward that degree than any other, and I was fortunate to meet and learn from some professors whose work continues to influence me today. I graduated and went on to earn a doctorate because if I'm going to be the first in my family to do something, I'm going to make damn sure I go the distance.

Now armed with several diplomas from prestigious universities,[4] all with the word "Psychology" on them, I've done a lot of different things as a psychologist. I've been a consultant, a professor, and even a therapist. I had to quit that last role because I got really sick of listening to people whine about their problems. Always with the yack, yack, yack, and I'd be thinking, *Shut up! You're not going to do what I'm going to tell you anyway. Give me your money and let's go home.* Actually, that's just a joke. I was never a therapist. I never wanted to go that route.

---

4 All of them packed away in a storage unit somewhere awaiting frames. At least I assume they are, as I haven't actually seen them in years. They may not be on the wall behind me, but I promise you they exist.

However, I did want to make people laugh. I'd always wanted to, but I never put any effort into doing so professionally until after I finished my doctorate degree. That was important for me to get first because I figured I needed a fallback plan in case my dream of being a comedian didn't work out. Most people chase the dream first; I chased my safety net first. It isn't how I'd recommend going about it,[5] but I like how everything worked out eventually.

The other reason I waited to start performing stand-up comedy was that I really had no idea how to get into it. As I mentioned, no one in my family had been to college, and certainly no one had attempted a career in entertainment, so I was clueless about how to start. Austin, where I went to college, is a great city for comedy, but I was too busy with schoolwork and other activities to get onstage. Then I went on to graduate school, which selfishly monopolized even more of my free time. Moving a few times in my early career didn't help either. Not to mention the near total lack of internet. Did you know that there was a time when you couldn't immediately find the answer to any random thought that popped into your head? You almost had to stumble onto things or forget about them.

I was living in San Francisco when I stumbled past a sign on my way home from work that advertised stand-up comedy classes, reminding me of my long neglected desire to be a comedian. I enrolled in the class as soon as I could, and within a week I was kicking myself for not starting sooner. I was shocked to learn that the barriers of entry for comedy are nonexistent—it was

5 I like to think that if I had started performing comedy in my teens, I would be famous by now. Sure, it would be more likely that I'd be waiting tables or trying to sell real estate, but this is my fantasy alternate universe, and I say I'm famous.

the making-a-living part that would prove to be difficult. This is why whenever anyone asks me what can you do with a degree in psychology, I always answer "comedian."

For a few years I was a solid presence in the San Francisco comedy scene, performing and developing my craft. I even opened up my own comedy club,[6] which allowed me to perform four nights a week and get better much faster than I would have if I'd had to rely on short open mic sets. Eventually being a comedian with a PhD in psychology led to public speaking opportunities and I started touring the country delivering humorous seminars on happiness and the health benefits of laughter.

And then I wrote a book.

During a seminar in Los Angeles, a talent agent asked me if I wanted to write one, and hell yes I did. A couple of weeks later, we were signing a fresh new contract over drinks at the Chateau Marmont on Sunset, because that's where all Hollywood contracts are signed. That book, *The Laughing Cure*,[7] remains a work that I am incredibly proud of and, unlike a lot of my earlier attempts at writing, rarely makes me cringe when I pick it up.

At the risk of spoiling that book for you, one of the primary benefits of humor is that it helps us manage stress. Humor also makes us happy, helps strengthen relationships, and has many physical benefits. However, as much as I loved sharing this message along with a few laughs, I realized that if I could help people learn

---

6 I recently learned that my club is mentioned in a footnote in Nina G. and O. J. Patterson's *Bay Area Stand-Up Comedy: A Humorous History* (Mt. Pleasant, SC: Arcadia Publishing, 2022), so here I am returning the favor.

7 Dr. Brian King, *The Laughing Cure: Emotional and Physical Healing: A Comedian Reveals Why Laughter Really Is the Best Medicine* (New York: Skyhorse, 2016).

how to better manage stress, that would really have an impact. The vast majority of all illnesses that we face in the modern world, both mental and physical, have a stress component. Not everything can be laughed off or joked about, and I became increasingly interested in stress management in general. This eventually led to my most recent book, *The Art of Taking It Easy*,[8] published toward the end of 2019. That book is a work I am truly proud of.

When *The Art* was released, it looked like it was positioned to do really well and take my career in new directions. I got a lot of good press, did a few local TV and radio interviews, and was even asked by the producers of a national talk show[9] to appear. I have written only two books at this point, and yet new writers ask me for advice all the time. The best advice I can give? Try not to publish your book just before a global pandemic. *The Art* came out a couple months prior to one of the most stressful periods of our lives, the COVID-19 pandemic. You may remember, people stopped buying things for a while, like books. Except toilet paper. People sure bought a lot of that for some reason. I joked with my publishers that we should have printed on two-ply. People would have boxes of my books in their closets. Read a page, use a page. "Hey, I gotta go to the can—will you pass me another copy of that book?" I still think that is a good idea. All kidding aside, everything was canceled for me: speaking tours, book signings, and media appearances. I lost my livelihood, and to make matters worse, this great book I had written was going to go relatively unnoticed. Of

8 Dr. Brian King, *The Art of Taking It Easy: How to Cope with Bears, Traffic, and the Rest of Life's Stressors* (New York: Apollo Publishers, 2019).

9 I won't name-drop the show, because it didn't happen, but my parents were big fans. Not getting on was probably more disappointing to them than to me.

course, underwhelming book sales were not the worst thing to happen during the pandemic.[10] That wasn't even the worst thing to happen to *me* during the pandemic, but it did hit me hard.

When the pandemic came to the United States, Sarah and I had been living on the road without a permanent residence for over five years, the last four with our daughter. We were a nomadic, vagabond family. We worked on the road and lived as we worked. When the government tells you to shelter at home and you don't have a home, what do you do? Thankfully we were in a position to go anywhere, and we chose to spend most of our time in Texas. I have always loved Texas, but after finishing college in Austin, I never thought I would move back. For the first time since leaving California, we had a place to call home for more than a few months. Despite everything, I think we all found it to be a refreshing change.

About six months into the pandemic, something really interesting happened. Maybe people were looking for ways to relieve their stress, maybe they were bored, or maybe they had completely run out of toilet paper and were super desperate, but people started buying my book. Especially in other countries! It became an international bestseller! Suddenly I started hearing from readers in places like Germany (*hallo!*), Brazil (*olá!*), and Poland (*dzień dobry!*). It has been amazing and has renewed my interest in being a writer.

So after writing books on humor and stress management, why turn my attention to weight management? Well, if you have read

---

10 I used to joke that with all that I lost during the pandemic, why couldn't some of it have been body weight?

those books, you probably can guess. If you haven't, another thing you should probably know about me is that throughout all of the experiences I have shared with you so far, I did everything with an extra person's worth of body weight attached to my frame. If I were on stage or TV right now, I wouldn't have to state the obvious, but since you are reading this, I'll put it as simply as I can: I am fat.

I'm a fat guy—and to paraphrase Janet Jackson, that's *Doctor* Fat Guy if you're nasty.[11] I'm not as fat as I used to be, thankfully. Over the past few years I've managed to lose about one hundred pounds. I still have a way to go before I get down to my goal weight, but that is badass. I look better, I feel incredible, and I can almost see my penis without a mirror. I hope that by the end of this book I'll be able to report, without lying to you, that I can see more of it. There must be more of it down there.

I may have my work cut out for me though. As soon as I got settled in Montreal, I hopped on a scale and saw that my recent tour and the road trip here had put about twenty pounds back on. The struggle is real, folks, the struggle is real.

11 But unlike Janet, I may let you call me "baby."

The Ship That Almost Passed Me in the Night

It is perfect timing that I am now at the part where I further introduce Sarah, as just yesterday we celebrated our seven-year anniversary. We share the day with the American Independence Day, which almost completely guarantees I will never forget it.[12] It also guarantees that every year for our special day, there will be fireworks. This time, since we're Americans living in Canada, we grabbed our passports and headed south to Plattsburgh, New York, with our daughter for a nice dinner before the show. I no doubt went way over my desired calorie count, probably setting back my progress even further, but it was an enjoyable, if not wildly debauched, evening, and I have successfully avoided my scale all day.

I don't remember meeting the woman whom I now refer to as my wife. For most guys, that might not be something they would want to openly admit, but my situation is a little different. When we met, I was just a few years into my career as a nationally touring public speaker and was giving a seminar on the topic of happiness in Gainesville, Florida, where she was living. At that time, I presented to thousands of people each year and talked to throngs of them every day. Looking back at my tour schedule for that year, I

12 It's in July, eh?

figured out that I had left Tallahassee the day before we met, presented in Gainesville, and traveled on to Tampa shortly after my seminar. My life moved fast then, and that tour was a whirlwind. I started the month in Texas, circled all around Florida, went on a cruise around the Caribbean, and ended back at my home in Los Angeles.

When the dust settled and I had a chance to sit back and take it easy, I went through my social media and reviewed the friend requests I received along the tour. Among them was one from an incredibly beautiful occupational therapist who lived in Gainesville. Her name was Sarah, and I could never have guessed the impact she would ultimately have on my life.

At the time, Sarah's profile photo was a side-by-side comparison of images of her before and after losing a substantial amount of weight. I thought she looked incredible in both shots. She had long red hair, which I have always been drawn to, bright eyes, a beautiful smile, and a perfect hourglass figure. I left a comment, "beautiful before, beautiful after," to which she replied, "Thank you Brian! I feel so much better though now! Much happier too!" As of this writing, that was eight years ago to the month, and it hardly reads like flirting, let alone the beginning of a long-term relationship.

The thing I didn't know about Sarah was that at the time of my seminar, she was thinking she could help me. I think she remembers it best, so I'll let her share her version of that day.

Not remembering when we met, Brian often makes up different jokes (depending on the company) about the day we met. There are probably about seven versions of our story milling around. One is about a cute woman in the back of the conference center getting up and repeatedly walking around, stretching, and trying to draw attention to herself. Apparently, I wasn't quite doing it right, as he didn't remember me later, but ironically enough that's exactly what I was doing that day. Sitting still has never been my style, and since I'd worked in busy hospitals and clinics for years, sitting still in a classroom-like setting for over six hours for a seminar was not my forte (nor, in my philosophy, what was best for my health).

Between stretching I would of course return to my seat, and luckily the seminar was far from boring. As a matter of fact, it was the best seminar I have attended to date. I listened intently, laughed, used what I heard to reflect on my own life, and took notes. Notes not only about the course material, but also general observations about seminar attendees and Dr. Brian King himself, including "poison berries, photography, and Luna." [More on why those are important later.] But one point of contention that stuck out in my mind and in my notes was this nonchalant statement he made, "Losing weight is easy! Eat less, move more." I kind of audibly and sarcastically chuffed, "Huh," and thought to myself, *It's not that easy.* I wrote down and underlined "NOT!"

> Having been through my own weight loss journey (and more than once, I might add) and having worked as an occupational therapist and a health coach in lifestyle redesign and weight loss, I knew that it wasn't that easy. Change isn't that easy, health is multifaceted, and human bodies are complicated and amazing. And then I thought to myself, *I'm going to help this guy. He seems like a tough nut to crack, but tenaciously I'm going to do it somehow.*
>
> Toward the end of the seminar, I walked in a polka-dot dress up to Brian, smiled, gave him my business card (which also included the before-and-after pic), asked a question about the course material, thanked him for the presentation, and the rest, as they say, is history. Well . . . sort of. There would be a lot of interaction points and "ships passing in the night" moments. What is it they say? It takes something like five interactions before a person remembers you.

At some point I started to notice Sarah on social media and began paying attention. We got to know each other a little through snarky comments, jokes, and the occasional interaction, and we even almost met up in San Francisco about a year after we first met, though that didn't work out—prompting Sarah to describe us as "ships passing in the night," a phrase I never really cared for. Then I had another seminar tour take me through Gainesville and was hoping to connect, but unfortunately Sarah was unable to attend. We finally met up socially about a year and a half after first following each other online, at a café in Tampa where she was temporarily working. I may not remember our first encounter, but trust me, I have a very vivid recollection of the second time we met.

Sarah and I share a mutual love of Cuban food—actually, most foods now that I think about it—and she suggested a nice casual spot called La Teresita. She arrived before me and ordered a drink. There was counter service as well as dining tables, and as I entered I saw her now-familiar, perfectly shaped hourglass figure perched on a stool at the counter. I think I fell in love in that moment, and I walked over to be as funny and charming as I could be so that she would do the same. It must have worked, because two days later she drove up to Gainesville to surprise me at a comedy show I was performing in.[13] Shortly after, I returned to Los Angeles and she took a contract in Boulder, Colorado, but in the months that followed, we were in touch more than ever, growing closer and closer despite the distance. By June I had made plans for a road trip to visit her in Colorado for the Fourth of July, for what we now refer to as our first date.[14]

Looking back, I wonder how many members of my audience had similar thoughts about helping me. That year, as I traveled the country, I was carrying around about 140 extra pounds of baggage strapped to the outside of my skeleton. It was like I was smuggling an extra person under my clothes to accompany me through life. And for what? So he could make my airplane seats seem smaller and prevent me from getting laid? When I was in college, I once

---

13 Sarah says, "I just really needed a good laugh so decided to be spontaneous and head to the show that night. I will admit the glazed-over, surprised look in his brown eyes was really cute that night as he scarfed down a much-needed preshow slice of pizza as treatment for hypoglycemia."

14 Prior to Sarah, I used to put geographical constraints on my dating life when I lived in various cities. For example, when I lived in San Francisco I had a strict "no bridge or tunnel" rule, and in Los Angeles I didn't want to date anyone east of Interstate 5 (and I really didn't like leaving West Hollywood). I broke a lot of rules to drive from Los Angeles to Boulder. Our official first date was at the Blues Traveler concert and fireworks show held in Red Rocks Amphitheatre.

got arrested in New York City when a buddy and I attempted to squeeze through a subway turnstile two at a time, but at least then we were trying to save a subway token by pretending to be a single dude. I had nothing to gain by lugging this stowaway on my body everywhere I went, yet there we were, flaunting our combined girth in front of audiences day after day, stuffed into an ever-tightening suit. I didn't look terrible, but my appearance was made ironic by the fact that my seminars then were all about how to change behavior and live a healthier life. I was a walking example of poor lifestyle choices, and I was telling people like Sarah how they could be healthier.

I may have inspired similar thoughts in others, but only Sarah chose to follow through and actually help improve my life. She had her work cut out for her too. She had to first convince me to pursue her halfway across the country, fall crazily in love with her, and have a child together. I don't work in health care, but that seems way beyond the usual call of duty for an occupational therapist.

FAT TALES

Bringing Sexy Back

I love Florida. On tour there sometime after my first encounter with Sarah, I did something so supercool, and funny, that the story made it into my stand-up act: I went swimming with manatees. If you don't know, manatees are large, docile aquatic mammals. I am sure you know what they are, but to make sure we are all on the same page, they are these giant-ass animals that weigh about a thousand pounds each and have tiny little eyes. They are cutest massive beasts you will ever encounter while exploring an environment clearly not intended for humans.

Manatees are a protected species, but there is one place in Florida, the Crystal River, where you are allowed to swim with them. So of course when my tour took me through that part of the country, I absolutely took advantage of the opportunity and booked a trip with one of the local manatee tour companies. Unfortunately, the first thing we were told we had to do was change into wet suits. Yeah, I'm not interested in putting on a wet suit and certainly wasn't back then, but Sean, the tour captain,[15] told me the water was too cold to go swimming without one, so I told him that I would just observe the manatees from the boat. At

15 Captain Sean is a very funny guy in his own right and would definitely be a great comedian had he chosen a different career. Book a tour with Mellow Mangrove Charters in Homosassa, Florida, and tell him I said hi.

this point I wasn't quite at my peak weight, but I was still clocking in somewhere above 350, and I assumed they wouldn't have a suit I could squeeze all of that into. I was wrong. I may have worn a 3XL shirt, but apparently 6XL was my wet suit size. It was the biggest size they had, but once they convinced me they had one that would fit me, I was like, OK, I guess I'm going in the water. Even at 6XL it was a little snug, so they helped me into it—well, put it on me—and it was an attractive look, me in a wet suit. Do you remember *Batman Returns*? I seriously looked like Danny DeVito playing the Penguin. Yep, I was bringing sexy back. Take that, Timberlake.

As soon as I was in the water, the manatees started approaching me. Seriously, I was only in the water for a few minutes when five or six giant manatees came straight up to me. My first response was to think, *Wow, this is incredible!* Then I looked around and noticed that none of the other divers were being approached and thought, *Wait a minute . . . in a wet suit, I kinda look like a manatee.*

I felt like they were saying, "Hey, who's the new guy? Welcome to our feeding grounds!"

It's weird that I had that thought, but I was in the water enjoying myself and floating around when they came over. If there is one thing I do well in water, it's float. I remember swimming lessons as a chubby kid when I struggled to learn the breaststroke, but the instructors told my parents, "He floats like a log!" You'll understand why then, when the guy on the boat asked if I wanted an additional floatie, I said, "No, I'm good. It's not like this body is going to sink."

Manatees are really neat creatures, and it's pretty cool when they come right up to you in the wild. They don't have any biting teeth, just ones for grinding, so they aren't very threatening. That doesn't stop them from trying to bite, though. They call it a manatee kiss, but I don't think they were trying to make out with me. Well, maybe one did hump my leg. But seriously, being in the water with them was a magical experience that I would recommend for anyone size 6XL and under.

And then the experience got a bit messy.

Here's the thing: I was wearing a wet suit. I was all snugged up in it and it was airtight. Just swimming around, having a good old time. Up until that point, I had never worn a wet suit before—surprise, I don't surf—and never having worn one, I didn't fully understand how they worked. I did, however, know that Captain Sean had encouraged me to wear it to keep warm, and that's all I thought it was doing, keeping me warm. But while I knew it was insulated, I didn't realize it was waterproof. Obviously it was keeping water away from my body, but I hadn't considered that enough to extend it to understanding that the wet suit would also keep in whatever bodily fluids I may have generated.

At this point you should know that I'm one of those guys who get in the water and very quickly after have to go. Surround me with a bunch of thousand-pound animals, and I'm definitely peeing. I couldn't hold back, but I thought it wouldn't be a big deal. When you pee in the ocean, you expect it's going to dissipate, or float away, and mingle with the rest of the water. Or maybe it'll make a little warm spot and you can call your brother over.

Urinate in a wet suit and it doesn't go away, at all. It stays there, in the suit attached to your body. Only you don't realize it because you are floating around with manatees enjoying this magical communion with nature. So I get out of the water and back on the boat. Everyone is having a good time, talking about the awesome experience we just shared. Next thing I know, I realize I've got a big pee bubble right around my pelvic region. I look down and I try to save face by saying it must be air, which would also be gross if you think about what air would be found near that part of my body, but it seemed less gross than admitting the truth. Captain Sean laughed. "There's always one!"

Slightly embarrassed, I went to the edge of the boat and manually pushed my pee bubble all the way down my leg and into the river. I then called my brother over and told him to check out the warm spot.

So I highly recommend that you swim with the manatees. Just don't pee in the wet suit.

A Promise I Intend to Keep

So why is a fat guy writing a book about how to lose weight? Yes, I have lost some of my excess weight, but I haven't lost all of it, and in fact I keep gaining back the same few pounds as I yo-yo myself through every special occasion.[16] So far I am down about 100 pounds from my peak, but I have probably lost about 250 pounds to get here. Weight loss books tend to be written by those who lose weight and keep it off, but here I am sitting on my bed, resting my laptop against my still-very-present belly while half tempted to go into the other room and raid my daughter's jar of hazelnut spread. I am very much a work in progress and may never fully achieve my goals. My story is common for sure. Most of us struggle to lose our extra weight, and very few of us are successful.

I am also someone with a degree in psychology, and as a person who has struggled with weight issues my entire life, I have always had an interest in the subject. I have done a bit of research on behavioral change, including what it takes to change the behaviors that contribute to body weight, and I have toured the country teaching people how to live healthier lives. Even if I haven't always modeled healthy choices myself, I understand what one should be doing and why so many of us have a hard time doing so.

I invited Sarah to have some input as well. As an occupational therapist, former life coach, art model, and someone who has had her own struggles with body weight, she will, I hope, provide some valuable insight to the discussion. At a minimum, she can keep me grounded when I go off on too many tangential stories or tell too many jokes, and generally keep me honest. She lives to correct me.

As an unencumbered bachelor I may have had an extremely indulgent and, at times, wild and crazy existence. However, when Sarah and I got together, she gave me life. More accurately, she gave me my life back. I was dying when I met her, and I knew it.

16 "I'm down two pounds! Let's celebrate with ice cream!" is probably a bad idea.

For years the consequences of routinely touring the country and indulging in all sorts of food and drink had been taking their toll. I could feel my health deteriorating, but I didn't really care. I was reckless. I took risks. Not unlike a rock star who develops a drug problem, I had a food problem. I've always had one, but touring gave me opportunities I'd previously never had. Every meal was in a restaurant in some new city, and I developed a talent for finding the biggest, baddest meals out there. I was definitely not a model of healthy living before I hit the road, but I was always able to keep my tendencies somewhat in check. At the bare minimum, when I lived in Los Angeles, I had a kitchen, and if I noticed my weight had gone up, I could focus on preparing lower-calorie meals to knock off the pounds. However, once I started traveling full-time for a living, it became harder and harder to maintain balance. With each tour, I would find myself eating and drinking my way across America. Some days my travel schedule was such that the only opportunity I had to enjoy myself was with a nice meal. I may have taught seminars by day, but at night I was still a comedian, and I was performing in clubs that offered me drinks in front of audience members who would sometimes do the same. I guess I'm lucky I never liked harder drugs.

I asked Sarah to add a story here about the early days of our relationship, as she can offer perspective.

> When Brian and I first started dating, he had already recognized he had a weight problem, and one night while giving one of our goodbye hugs he asked me to wrap my arms around him and try to remember where my arms met each

> other. He said the next time we saw each other, he wanted my hands to be able to reach closer together. However, as time passed, my hands did not get any closer. In fact, they started to get farther apart.
>
> Later in our relationship, we planned an adventurous trip together to Australia. I was six months pregnant, and many of our friends found it absurd that we'd decided to travel through the Australian outback in 104°F (40°C) summer weather and pictured me waddling miserably in the heat. However, it would not be me doing the waddling. I will never forget the day we arrived in Byron Bay and decided to go to the lighthouse. There was a small, short path where you could go out and stand to look out from the most eastern point of Australia. It didn't look very far away at all, and naturally I wanted to go and check it out. Brian, however, was short of breath, complained of knee pain, and his back felt so sore that he had to stop frequently, and so he refused to walk with me. It was disappointing to say the least, but more importantly I remember walking back from the point by myself, sad and worried. I was wondering with real concern if the baby I was carrying was going to have a father to help raise her.

Even with Sarah's help, and despite all her effort, my health continued to deteriorate. She could only do so much. As a health-care professional, Sarah always urged me to see a doctor, but I would refuse. Partly out of arrogance, but also due to the fact I knew all my problems stemmed from my need to lose weight. My attitude was, Why should I pay someone to tell me what I already know? So

I refused to go. I figured that I had managed to lose weight before and I could do it again, although I clearly wasn't managing.

When Sarah found out she was pregnant, I was in the worst condition I had ever been in. She finally convinced me to get a checkup before our daughter was born. I knew I was in rough shape, but I had no idea the extent of the damage I had done to myself until Sarah kicked my ass into an urgent care clinic. After removing my shoes, because everyone knows that heavy shoes are the real scale tipper, I weighed in at exactly four hundred pounds.[17] I was blown away. I knew I had gotten heavy, but gorilla heavy? Never before in my life had I seen such a high number on a scale. I was ashamed of how badly I had let myself go. And that was the beginning of the checkup—there was more news to follow.

I also found out that my blood pressure was dangerously high. That was not surprising given all the extra fat I was carrying, but it was painfully ironic given that I had been earning a living by teaching people how to manage stress for several years—a tool that can help keep blood pressure in check. I was also told that my legs and feet were swollen.

My health issues were definitely a concern, but apparently they had not been reason enough to motivate real change. According to Sarah:

> The first and most important question is the why. What is your motivation for wanting to lose weight and get healthy? Maybe you want to fit into a pair of new jeans and look

---

17 I have never publicly stated that number before and only shared it with Sarah and a few close friends. Even writing it now, committing it to publication, feels super weird.

better (that's fine). Maybe you want to be present for your kid's college graduation (better answer). Honestly, there is no wrong answer. It's always good to get healthy. Any excuse will do, but a really good reason is even better.

The stronger the reason for the motivation and the deeper, more meaningful, and more wellness oriented it is, the more likely you will be to stick with your weight loss plan. Why again? Because you have something to remind yourself of when the going gets hard at 3 a.m., when you are tired and may not be making the best choices while watching QVC, adding items to your Amazon shopping cart, or ransacking your cupboard. Because you have something stronger pulling you up to take a break from your desk or away from your television set to go take that afternoon walk.

The primary reason I am writing this book is that five years ago I made a promise to a very special person in my life, our daughter, Alyssa, when she was born. I held her in my arms for the first time, looked into her beautiful eyes, and promised her that Daddy was going to get healthier.

And I'm trying. I'm trying really hard even though it has been a constant struggle. It's been five years, and I've lost about one hundred pounds, give or take whatever I gained yesterday.

The Best Things About Losing One Hundred Pounds

In no specific order, the best things about losing one hundred pounds are:

- I feel ~~great~~ *fantastic.*
- I can walk for greater distances without pain or discomfort and without loss of breath.
- I can go on carnival rides with my daughter.
- I can sit on the floor with my legs crossed and play Barbies with my daughter.
- I have more energy onstage both as a comedian and public speaker.
- I no longer require a seat belt extension on an airplane.
- I look better in (and can fit into) my clothes again.
- Everyone who hasn't seen me in a long time tells me how good I look.
- Sex is better, and my sex drive has increased.
- Sarah lets me be on top again.

2

Two Simple Methods

There is a story that I often tell about how one day at one of my seminars someone asked me if I had any tips on how to lose weight. It was a common question; I assume because I would often speak about behavioral change and use examples pertaining to food, but . . . really? Did I look like the guy you ask for weight loss tips? I looked like that guy's before-picture. I looked like the guy you ask for restaurant suggestions, and I could definitely offer those, but if I had any answers worth a damn about weight loss, I doubt I would have been carrying around so much extra mass under my clothes.

Holding back my tendency to reply with sarcasm, I said that this was actually a subject that I had done a fair amount of research on. I shared that, according to the literature, there were two simple methods that were scientifically proven to result in lower body weight. Each of these methods was supported by tons of data and observations. In fact, I continued, if a person could implement just one of these methods, they were almost guaranteed to lose weight. With both methods, the weight would come right off. With an eager look, she asked me, "Well, what are they?"

"The first method is simple," I said. "You're going to have to eat a lot less."

"Oh." She seemed disappointed. "What's the second method?"

I told her that the second method is a little more complicated but still relatively simple and shared, "You're going to have to exercise a lot more."

"Oh, so that's it? Diet and exercise?" She seemed very underwhelmed. She then said, "Yes, but what *else* can I do? I hate exercising and I love food!"

Diet and exercise being key is no big mystery, and for the vast majority of us, all we need is to make some changes to those two behaviors. We all know how to lose weight, and yet so many of us (myself included) have such a hard time implementing this knowledge. Hell, I've known how to lose weight my entire life, and I've also been overweight for most of my life. How do you eat less and exercise more? That's the hard part.

What's that? Sarah looks like she has something to say. . . .

> I actually laughed out loud and said "Not!" the first time I heard Brian make the statement that all it takes to lose weight is to eat less and exercise more. Why? Because in my experience, weight loss is a lot more multifaceted than that. I know that in essence he's right, but it's almost insulting to put it that simply, as if he were saying that weight loss is easy.

> To me, weight loss is a lot like pain management. We all want to take some magic pill and have our pain go away. We also want a pill that will help us lose weight quickly. Just taking a pill for this, something as easy as pushing a button, would be nice, wouldn't it? Done! Poof! But in my many years as a clinician, I've learned that oftentimes pain doesn't easily go away. Its treatment may include pills or creams, even things you smoke, or it may take surgery or physical and occupational therapy treatments, including exercise, strengthening, stretching, and contracture management, or modalities such as electrical stimulation, laser therapy, and diathermy. Treatment may also include acupuncture, deep breathing techniques, visualization, reframing, stress management, dietary change, and, dare I say, weight loss.
>
> So diet and exercise, yes, absolutely essential—but not only those. Then what else? As an occupational therapist and as a health coach who's dealt with lifestyle redesign, I always approach my clients first by getting to know more about them with an interview that includes questions about medical and personal history and a lot about their lifestyle and habits. After that, we can begin formulating a game plan that works for them.

I guess another option is being content with an overweight and unhealthy body. For the longest time, I convinced myself that I didn't need to lose weight. Although I was carrying more than I needed (clearly preparing for a famine that never came), I believed I was in fairly good health and lived a happy life. I never seemed to have problems finding women to date. Lucky for me,

I've found that women generally find brains and humor attractive qualities in a mate and are sometimes willing to overlook the lack of abdominal muscles. Hell, I managed to convince Sarah to fall in love with me, and she's a freaking model.

If you've made it this far then you have probably picked up on the fact that in this book I will not be claiming to have all the answers to weight loss, or any that you don't already know. If I had some special technique to share, some secret method or set of mystery behaviors, I would be writing this in between fashion shows and photo shoots because, duh, clearly, I would be a model.

Sorry to disappoint, but to paraphrase Glinda the good witch,[18] you've always had the power to lose the weight. For most of us, we are going to have to eat less and exercise more. It's simple, but it ain't easy. If it were easy, I would have already achieved my goal and celebrated the birth of my daughter by doing one-arm pull-ups while high-fiving doctors in the delivery room. Instead, this is the only weight loss book I am aware of that is written by someone who is currently obese. I'm not going to pretend to be some great and all-powerful wizard like in Oz,[19] but I can tell you how I am working toward my goals, and I can share what has worked for others. Maybe this will be inspiring, or perhaps even motivating, but ultimately each of us is going to need to adopt a healthier mindset and figure out how to eat less and exercise more. Hopefully, we can have a few laughs along the way.

---

18 I kinda feel like I don't need to cite this, but old habits die hard, so: *The Wizard of Oz*, directed by Mervyn LeRoy, Victor Fleming, King Vidor, George Cukor, Norman Taurog, and Richard Thorpe (California: Metro-Goldwyn-Mayer, 1939).

19 He turned out to be a fake anyway.

CONSULTING THE EXPERT

Bodybuilder Andrew Ginsburg

Diet and exercise. It can't really be that simple, can it?

For most of us, the answer is yes. For a small percentage of us, the answer is yes but. . . . Regardless of our special circumstances, losing weight means using more energy than we take in.

After my first book was published, I started to receive review requests from other authors and publishers. I guess the logic was that because I wrote a book, I must now be an expert on reading books. Whatever my opinion is worth, one book that came my way was *Pumping Irony*[20] by comedian and bodybuilder Andrew Ginsburg. I remember thinking, *What an appropriate match. Here I am, a psychologist and comedian who uses humor to teach lessons supporting mental health, and there's Andrew, a personal trainer and comedian who uses humor to teach lessons of physical health. Man, I hope it's good.*

Thankfully it was, and I still frequently recommend it to people. Through correspondence, Andrew and I became acquainted with one another, and I saw a lot of parallels in our lives, and not just in performing comedy and writing books. We are both originally from New York, and we both became fathers around

20 A quick Google search informed me that Andrew's book's title is not the only one starting with the words "Pumping Irony," so please make sure you check out: Andrew Ginsburg, *Pumping Irony: How to Build Muscle, Lose Weight, and Have the Last Laugh* (New York: Skyhorse, 2017).

the same time. However, one of us looks better in a Speedo than the other. I'll let you ponder that visual and decide which one as I share my interview with him.

Brian: Could you tell me a bit about your career?

Andrew: If we are solely speaking about fitness, I was a tennis player growing up and tennis got me into college, where I played at Boston University. I started lifting weights to improve my tennis game and enjoyed the workouts as much as the tennis. As my body grew stronger and my physique developed, I decided to compete in a teenage bodybuilding competition. I did my first contest at eighteen and my most recent one two weeks ago at forty-two.[21]

Brian: How far have you made it in the world of bodybuilding?

Andrew: I've won three titles: Mr. New England, Mr. Staten Island, and Mr. Long Island, and I came in fourth in the World Natural Bodybuilding Federation's championships. Natural bodybuilding is kind of an oxymoron, but I've never taken steroids, which are pretty widespread in the sport. So I've done pretty well.

Brian: You started being highly physically active at an early age with tennis and then bodybuilding. At what point did you become a comedian?

Andrew: In college, right around the time I started bodybuilding. I met this guy, Teddy Bergeron—a legendary Boston comic—and he kind of took me under his wing. So I did them in tandem and was a personal trainer and comedian. It was a weird combination; one is late night and one starts early in the morning.

Brian: It sounds like almost the opposite of how I did it. I'd

21 He's also younger, but whatevs.

eat and drink all day, and then do comedy. Comedians generally don't exhibit the healthiest behaviors, so it's an interesting combination to see in you. There's a lot of drugs, a lot of alcohol, a lot of indulgences in comedy. And you worked as a personal trainer?

Andrew: I've been doing personal training since I was about twenty-one. I've always been into exercise and stand-up comedy, and never with a lapse in either of those.

Brian: The book I'm writing is all about weight loss, including my own personal weight loss, as I'm trying to lose weight and become a healthier person. Basically, to be more like you. What tips do you have for people who are trying to manage their weight?

Andrew: I think it comes down to meal preparation. No one ever mentions that, but it's the most important element to weight loss. If you know what you are eating at your next meal ahead of time, there is no guesswork and no real opportunities to overeat. If you open the refrigerator and you don't know what the hell you are having, you are more likely to grab something that is not ideal for weight loss or even weight maintenance. I think it's underrated how important meal preparation is. If you know what your breakfast, lunch, and dinner are going to be the night before, it is going to make it a hell of a lot easier. It's definitely not as interesting or exciting. People like to say, "What will we have for dinner?" But if you want to reach your goal, meal prep is everything. I would put that as number one above anything else, what you put in your mouth. The exercise is cute, but a bad diet with exercise is not going to get you in shape.

Brian: What sort of foods would you recommend?

Andrew: Everyone is different. Obviously there is no

one-size-fits-all answer, but I would start with a high-protein diet, eating carbohydrates in the morning and cutting them out as the day goes on. It's really based on your activity level: you don't need carbohydrates if you're at home with your kid doing math from books or watching television, but if you are going to be getting some exercise or are going to be outside doing yard work, then you are going to need carbohydrates. Otherwise, you don't. I don't like that keto stuff because sometimes you need carbohydrates. Try to figure it out by eating different foods and seeing how you react and what your energy levels are. Some people work really well with fats and other people with carbohydrates, but you don't need both. I would experiment with food and see what your body loses weight better with. Some people have to really reduce carbs, while others don't have to. Some work better with higher fat and super-low carbs.

I would break it down to three or four meals a day depending on your energy needs and level of hunger. I believe in sustainability in every sense. If you can't eat the same way or do a certain kind of workout for the rest of your life, it's not going to work.

Brian: That makes a lot of sense. Regarding exercise, I know you're a bodybuilder, but for those of us who are wanting to increase activity and maybe lose a little bit of weight but not necessarily bulk up, are there any particular exercise routines that you recommend?

Andrew: Any cardiovascular exercise that you enjoy. A bike ride or whatever it is you like. Make sure you're burning calories and getting your heart rate up for at least twenty to thirty minutes per day. You know what the best workout is? It's the one you're going to do. If you're going to do weight lifting, the most effective exercises are the ones where your torso travels through space, like with squats, lunges, and crunches.

To work a number of muscles at once, you'll want to do compound movements. People like bicep curls, but they only work a tiny portion of your body, whereas a lunge engages your core and works your legs. Your legs and back are the biggest muscles for weight loss, so focus on those areas. Squats and lunges, anything where you are standing up, are obviously better than sitting. Whatever workout you're doing, it's all movement. As long as you are doing something, it's going to be fine.

Brian: We've talked a bit about what we eat and exercise, and before the interview, we were talking about a trifecta of things that we should pay attention to in regard to health. Would you like to touch on that too?

Andrew: I think there are three parts: exercise, nutrition, and sleep. No one ever talks about sleep, but like water, nobody gets enough of it. And if you don't sleep enough, your body is going to store fat, increase your cortisol level, and also be more inclined to eat carbohydrates. It's going to lead to eating ice cream and not egg whites or eggs (I love the yolks[22]). Then there's exercise, of course, partnered with nutrition; but if you were to weigh them, I'd say nutrition is King. No pun intended.[23]

We're basically a heap of food. If you see someone, you have no idea how much they exercise, but you have a decent idea of

---

22 I'm still not sure why every movie with a workout montage shows people slurping down raw eggs. Are they somehow more nutritious straight out of the shell? I am convinced it just looks cool on camera.

23 And yet, given the name Dr. Brian King, the pun was very much taken!

what they're eating, whether it's nutrient-dense or not.

Brian: That is such a great way to put it. I always think of us as big bags of meat, but I never think of us as a walking stack of food. It's very true.

Andrew: We *are* a heap of food. I look at somebody and I get a pretty good idea of what they eat. If someone is heavy, there's probably quite a bit of processed foods and maybe alcohol in their diet. Obviously genetics play a role, but healthy eating will help anyone get in shape.

Brian: With your personal training clients, what do you see as their biggest obstacle to achieving their goals?

Andrew: Meal preparation. Some clients were getting results, but I knew they would be sped up with better eating, so I gave them lots of options for each meal based on their preferences. You don't have to have chicken breast at every meal. There's a lot of protein sources: eggs, chicken, salmon, turkey, protein shakes . . . If you're vegetarian it's harder, but there's quinoa and other stuff. Late-day carbs also tend to be a problem. All the damage happens after 4 p.m.

Brian: As you know, I'm the father of a five-year-old girl, and I've also been overweight my entire life. One of my major concerns is raising a fit child. Do you have any recommendations for raising children, especially in today's world with the difficulties that we have in maintaining healthy lifestyles?

Andrew: It's really hard, because I'm eating the chicken breast and the broccoli but my kids are like any other kids. They want mac and cheese and fruit snacks. They want the peanut butter crackers and the cheese crackers. I'm kind of honoring that because they're kids, but I definitely put healthy choices in front of them. I tell them certain foods are muscle foods, like eggs, chicken, and fruit, and ultimately set a good example with my own eating.

Brian: I made my daughter a promise when she was very young. I told her I was going to get healthier for her and that one day we could run together. We're still not in a state where I can run a lot, but I'm definitely a lot healthier and a lot more physically active with her, that's for sure.

Andrew: You'll get there. Keep in mind that as parents over forty, it's crucial that we don't get injured in the gym with bad form or weights that are too heavy. Same for long-distance running. Higher reps with lighter weights and perfect form will keep us fit for chasing our kids around.

FAT TALES

That Doctor Comedian

When I am traveling I usually avoid chain restaurants, but I went to an Outback Steakhouse for the first time recently. Have you been to one? They advertise it as the Australian-themed steakhouse, but let me tell you, there was not a damn thing Australian on that menu. I was hoping for a kangaroo steak, maybe some fried emu strips, or a koala burger. There was none of this. It's regular food. They used to run commercials with the slogan "No rules, just right," and it was even printed on their menu. Really? If you don't have any rules, then how about I don't pay for this meal? How about I don't wear pants? How about you serve me up some koala meat like I wanted? They are cute animals; I bet they taste adorable. They should change that slogan to "Outback Steakhouse: Australian for Applebee's."[24]

By the way, during the trip Sarah and I took to Australia when she was a few months pregnant with Alyssa, we took two of our Australian friends to the Outback Steakhouse in Brisbane. Let's just say that they were not impressed, though the menu at that location is a bit more Australian than you find in the States, and our friends thought the "onion thing" was awesome.

As a comedian, I never broke into any level of public awareness. I remember speaking with my first publicist, who asked me, "I'm sorry, I don't follow comedy. Are you a famous comedian?" Part of being famous is not having to tell people that you're famous. Despite not being famous, I have performed in a lot of clubs and at festivals across the United States, Canada, and even Australia, where I definitely did not use the Outback Steakhouse bit. I moved to Los Angeles to try to get famous, but I discovered I liked traveling on the road more and missed a lot of auditions, so here I am.

One thing I have always loved about stand-up comedy is that anyone, regardless of their physical appearance, can be funny. While the acting and music worlds tend to reward performers

---

24 You remember those Foster's Beer "How to speak Australian" commercials, right?

who are young and thin, comedy is more inclusive. Those who make it big are often younger and thinner, but there are a lot of fat comedians. When I started performing, it seemed that there were tons[25] of comics who shared my physical characteristics, which is why I adopted "Dr. Brian King" as my stage name. Before I became a comedian, I never used my title, but I thought it helped me stand out from all the other overweight white male comedians out there. It worked too. On several occasions I have been stopped on the street by people who've asked if I am "that doctor comedian."

John DeKoven, who was the owner of Bunjo's Comedy Club[26] in Dublin, California, once put together a showcase of comedians called "The Big Boys of Comedy," with me as the headliner. I didn't get that gig because I was young and thin. I am still surprised our combined mass didn't collapse the stage the night we performed. As it happens, Bunjo's was located in a Chinese restaurant right next to an Outback Steakhouse, which is where that bit came from in the first place.

When I got serious about losing weight, the thought crossed my mind about how it would affect my comedy. Could I still use some of my fat jokes? Would I even still be funny? It seems like a ridiculous concern, as humor isn't tied to fat, but I did develop my sense of humor in part as a means to overcome my weight. It isn't that unreasonable to at least ponder the question. I have seen performers significantly alter their body shape and struggle to

25 Yes, the pun is intended.

26 Unfortunately no longer operating.

maintain their audience.[27] I won't mention any names, because I don't want to say anything potentially negative about someone's weight loss, but I have observed that when a comedian rose to fame as an overweight person—and overweight is the image I have of them in my head—it can be a little hard to accept the more fit version when I see them onstage.

Thankfully, I am not yet famous. Maybe I would be if I had a better publicist.

Yeah, I might have to scrap a few jokes here and there, and alter my stage persona a bit, but ultimately my daughter needs a healthy daddy more than the world needs to hear my jokes about food. And by the way, I've lost five more pounds since I began writing this book!

CONSULTING THE EXPERT

Chef Suzi Gerber

Early in my career I took a job in Pittsburgh. Prior to my interview, I had never been to Pittsburgh before, but as I drove in, I realized it would be a great place to call home for a few years. The hilly

27 Here is a nice article on the subject: Hollie McKay, "Do Fat Comedians Lose Some Giggles When They Lose the Jiggles?" (Fox News, April 8, 2016), https://www.foxnews.com/entertainment/do-fat-comedians-lose-some-giggles-when-they-lose-the-jiggles.

landscape reminded me of San Francisco, and the urban architecture reminded me of Gotham City as portrayed in *Batman* comics.[28] There was a postindustrial feel to some neighborhoods and the city overall that gave it an interesting character. Although it wasn't the first city to come to mind when I was thinking about my career after graduate school, Pittsburgh was ripe with potential. I met a lot of creative people in the Burgh: artists, filmmakers, musicians, and actor types. It was the kind of city that attracted them by being both affordable and somewhat inspiring. It was in this context that I first met Chef Suzi Gerber.

Suzi was an artist with the brain of a scientist, and I was a scientist with the heart of an artist, so I think it is clear why we hit it off. We worked on a few projects together and became good friends. She knew me before I became a comedian, and I knew her before she became a chef (and, later, a doctoral candidate). Eventually we would both leave our home in southwestern Pennsylvania for other cities, but over the years we've managed to stay in touch, and as we share an affinity for many of the same places, we even bump into each other all over the world. Most recently, Sarah and I enjoyed a vegan dinner at Suzi's restaurant in Boston. It was so delicious that I barely noticed the lack of animal products.

I toyed with veganism in college, mainly for weight loss, but I also remember feeling more energetic and healthier overall. When Suzi's cookbook, *Plant-Based Gourmet*,[29] came out, I was considering a return to that lifestyle and thought, *Who better to*

---

28 Coincidentally, years later Pittsburgh would play Gotham City in *The Dark Knight Returns* (2012).

29 Suzi Gerber, *Plant-Based Gourmet: Vegan Cuisine for the Home Chef* (New York: Apollo Publishers, 2020).

serve as my expert for the diet portion of the two simple methods than Chef Suzi? She is almost always an incredibly busy person, and as I write this she is currently in graduate school finishing her PhD, but thankfully she was able to fit me in.

Brian: What should I list as your occupation now? I want to call you a chef, but I know you are more than that.

Suzi: Technically I am a behavior scientist and a nutrition scientist. Either or both.

Brian: All right, that's the angle I'm going with. First of all, you have had your own struggle with weight loss. Can you tell me a bit about that?

Suzi: I was always overweight as a child. Most of the people in my family are overweight. I think the dieting process for me started as a very young child. I've tried a bunch of different things over the years. I was very notably a junk food vegan in the nineties and went straight from that to the Atkins diet.

Brian: You were a vegan but then started a very meat-oriented diet?

Suzi: My family doctor sat me down with my mom and said, "She's a teenager and she's never going to lose weight on the diet she's on now. She's never going to be healthy unless she eats meat." I was maybe a sophomore or junior in high school, and overnight I went from being vegan to being on Atkins. All I ate was meat, like sliced meat and sliced cheeses. I was always very athletic and involved in a lot of endurance activities, so I had really good muscle density and strength, but I was always overweight. Then in my early twenties I developed a very serious chronic illness. My ability to function and do some of those athletic activities was strongly impacted. I wasn't able to do yoga anymore. My doctors told me that I wasn't allowed to carry more than the weight of my laptop for risk of injury.

For about five years in my late twenties, I was chronically ill and very overweight, probably the heaviest I've ever been in my life. During that time, I must have tried everything under the sun to lose weight. I was super health conscious, and I would only eat organic food and tons of fruit and vegetables. I was living in Manhattan and I was quite sick. Manhattan is a food paradise. You can literally live any way in the world in Manhattan, but nothing worked. I looked through everything and I read everything. One day I stumbled upon something that said there had been a lot of clinical trials and observational studies that showed that people could reverse chronic illnesses similar to mine with a vegan diet.

I was vegan in the nineties when it was cool, so I decided I was going to give it another shot. I was like, this is going to be easy, I know how to be vegan. My husband at the time was a Midwest meat-and-potatoes guy. I was shocked he went along for the ride with me on this. He was pretty heavy himself. We lost a ton of weight really fast, within a month. I was off all of this medication that I had been on for years. I was totally asymptomatic and the weight kept coming off and I was able to do all the sporty stuff I used to do.

It was life-changing, and it was really interesting to me because I was living a very different life then. I was more involved in visual arts at that time, and I was like, man, this is where it's at: food and health. This is what changes people's lives. It changed my life. So I dove in and tried to learn more about what the evidence base said about it. Entering the cooking world was a little bit more accessible to me at the time. I wanted to learn how to sustain this way of life. I was a big foodie. Again, Manhattan was a food playground for me, and I didn't want to give that up entirely. I discovered this whole world of how possible it was to eat gourmet as a vegan and how possible it was to be healthy and gourmet and be really experimental. It's only gotten more interesting and diverse from there.

Brian: As you know, I'm writing a book, which means I have to sit at a computer for what seems like all the time. Writing is not a task that involves a great deal of physical activity, but I make an effort. After I complete a section, I'll tell my daughter that we have to go for a walk because Daddy needs to burn some calories. As much as I try, it's hard to stay active, so I'd like to get your opinion. From a nutritional perspective, how should I structure my eating so that I can lose weight?

Suzi: There are really a couple of different ways that I would tell almost anybody, but I've known you for what feels like fucking forever at this point, so I might tailor my opinions for you. I think a really important part of weight loss is understanding that there are biological ways that everybody can lose weight, and then there are ways that with your lifestyle might work for you. I can tell you about the wonders of a vegan diet. I can tell you about the wonders of eating more fruits and vegetables and whole grains. We hear all of these things all the time, and I do strongly believe that that's the best way, but the best diets are the diets that you stick to. The best diet is the diet you can follow.

You have to make a series of compromises in your life. That

can be meal to meal, month to month, or year to year. That's how I like to encourage people to think about it. Sometimes we think every meal is an opportunity to eat the most delicious thing available to us at the restaurant we're at or in the grocery store. I usually tell people, maybe reorient that thinking first. Not every meal has to be the most exciting meal ever. But you definitely should not approach every meal like I'm going to choke this awful thing down because I have to. That's not going to get you very far. That'll get you through a crash diet for a month, maybe, and then leave you worse off at the end of it.

The research is very clear that the more often you try and fail at a diet, the less weight you'll lose and the less you'll be able to keep it off. I think everybody should take a pretty honest inventory with themselves about what they are willing to give up and where the compromises lie. Some of those compromises are going to be about goals; losing weight fast and keeping weight off are not the same thing. Maybe you don't want to give up meat or maybe you don't want to give up ice cream, but be honest with yourself.

If you want to lose weight, you might lose a lot of it really fast and then completely change your strategy. That one actually works really well for me. A lot of the popular diets have induction periods. I think induction periods are really well supported by the literature. Think about a one-month plan and that plan has a really intense month where you have to bite the bullet and get through it. Let's say you drop ten to twenty pounds in that month. They usually tell you not to try to lose more than two and a half pounds a week. So ten pounds in a month is totally achievable.

Once you get past that point, you'll say, "The month that I just did, eating twelve hundred calories a day and not eating my favorite foods, is not how I intend to live the rest of my life, because nobody succeeds living that way. But it got me to where I am, and now I want to set some different goals."

Maybe your second goal is putting on some muscle, because that will help you in the long run too. I usually say it's like cut, then gain, then maintain. I've done this with myself a few times. I like to do a vegan keto for two months. I lose a lot of weight really fast, fifteen or twenty pounds. That is focused on cutting down fat mass, and after I want to make sure I'm bringing up my protein a little bit and bringing up my resistance exercise activities, so that I'm putting on lean mass, because that will increase my metabolism. My appetite levels will naturally reduce. Then I shift to a moderate carb, moderate protein, moderate fat diet. I go into maintenance, which is accurately assessing what the caloric need is to maintain your ideal body weight.

Brian: I was vegan twice in my life. The first time, I lost a lot of weight and then ended up eating nothing but peanut butter and jelly sandwiches. The other time was right before the pandemic.

Suzi: I think you came to my restaurant that second time.

Brian: Yes, I was up in Boston and ate at your restaurant. I was strict, and as I was traveling, I found I was eating all these plant-based hamburgers. They may be a great meat substitute, but they are certainly not low calorie or all that healthy. I felt as if veganism was very hard to maintain on the road.

Suzi: There are different goals. I think goals are a really important part of the conversation, because if your sole goal is to be vegan, you could eat potato chips for breakfast, lunch, and dinner. Potato chips are probably the single food most associated with obesity in the United States.

There are various kinds of veganism. I think that the beauty of a vegan diet is that you can find a diet that works for you, whatever your other goals are. If your goals are ecological sustainability or personal health or animal welfare or a combination, you can find it. But you're right that substituting a vegan burger for an animal-based burger is a modest dietary improvement at best. A burger is a burger.

I don't say vegan because it has a health halo. I say vegan because it is an accurate assessment of my diet, but it's not where the buck stops. I will often eat dinners that are 50 percent broccoli. I could just as easily have dinners that were 50 percent french fries.

Brian: I was fully aware that I wasn't eating health food when I was eating those burgers. The problem was this lifestyle of being on the road. It was a convenient and easy way to stay vegan while I was traveling.

Suzi: I also think that there's a difference between vegan, or any diet, for weight loss and any diet for health. I think this is often lost in the sauce when people talk about weight loss, because you can eat nothing but fat and still lose weight.

Brian: I want to talk a little about your cookbook. Where did that come from?

Suzi: The inspiration for that was very much about trying to share the joy of gourmet vegan, cooking with people, because as a spoiled vegan who cut her adult vegan teeth in Manhattan, I had everything available to me. I really do think that when you have exposure to what's possible in veganism, when it's not just plant-based burgers or mac and cheese or french fries to choose from, it's more possible for people to imagine their life on those foods. They are the foods that I enjoyed and knew would be missed sorely when I left Manhattan. For me, that cookbook was filling a gap, making people aware that vegan food could be gourmet and delicious. The book is not at all health-focused. I think there's plenty of healthy stuff in it, but there's also a lot of pastry in there. There's plenty of sugar and coconut oil too.

I think that most people have an automatic assumption that plant-based is restrictive, but actually, in the average American diet, people eat the same ten to thirteen things over and over again. When you go plant-based, I feel like there's a whole other culture involved. So all these foods become super normal. I think hundreds of new fruits and vegetables and plants and things to do with them just became normal in my life.

You know, I think your peanut butter and jelly thing seems almost like an executive function issue. Like I don't want to make decisions anymore, and this is here and I know I like it and I'm just going to go for it. I think that a lot of people, regardless of whether they're vegan or not, fall into those slumps. Even chefs fall into these slumps. I got to the point where I am so busy every morning that my breakfast most mornings is a block of baked tofu. It is perfectly palatable, but not exciting. And it has some of those hallmarks of cutting back on decision-making. For me it's like I'm going to save my executive functioning for other, more important things, because the rest of my day is data analysis.

3

Studies of Eating and Screwing

I am not an expert in fitness like Andrew Ginsberg, or an expert in nutrition like Chef Suzi Gerber. In fact, I hesitate to call myself an expert in anything, but I do know a few things about human behavior. I suppose I have always been interested in why we do what we do. As a human being myself, I have always observed, interpreted, and attempted to understand my own behavior and that of others. In this sense, every person is an amateur psychologist.

As I mentioned, I went to college at the University of Texas at Austin, a well-ranked institution of higher learning and an awesome place to go to college. I've joked that when my daughter is old enough, she can go to any college she wants, as long as it is UT Austin. Much like the campus of McGill University here in Montreal, UT's is in the middle of the city and surrounded by a vibrant and stimulating scene. It is a beautiful, collegiate-looking university filled with great architecture and public art, and I was lucky to attend. And I do mean lucky—it was dumb luck really. I know that a lot of prospective students research various schools and programs, and maybe visit a few campuses, before making a decision about where to apply, but I did nonc of that. I was living in Austin when I finished high school and simply applied to the local college. I did no research and never considered other options. I picked my college because it was local. At the time I had no idea how different educational experiences could be. I did not start college specifically to earn a degree in psychology, but eventually I found my way to that department as my interests developed over time. The UT psych-department faculty included some very prominent researchers in the relatively new field of evolutionary psychology. Of course, hindsight is twenty-twenty, but I think I was lucky to attend such a university, and I was lucky to have studied with some very influential thinkers. I was at the right place at the right time.

I have always been overweight, and therefore I have always, to some degree, been interested in weight-related issues. However, it was a psychology class at UT that first led me to think about them with more than casual observation. The class had an unusual title, something like "Substance Abuse: Food and Alcohol," which was intriguing, but more importantly, it fit my schedule. From the first day, the professor, Dr. Devendra Singh,[30] impressed me with his use of humor, stories about elephants and India, and the fact that at the end of each day he would reward students who answered questions correctly with a fresh fig. It was

30 In preparing for this book, I was saddened to learn that unfortunately Dr. Singh passed away in 2010. It would have been wonderful to get to talk with him again.

one of the few classes in my academic career that I made a point to never miss, and I frequently visited Dr. Singh during office hours.[31] I never got a fig, but the information he covered and his eye-opening theories changed how I view the world and later inspired my own research.

Dr. Singh was best known for his work on the importance of fat distribution in determining physical attractiveness. Fat distribution is expressed as waist-to-hip ratio[32] (WHR) and is simply measured by taking the circumference of the waist and dividing by the circumference of the hips. If a person's hips are wider than their waist, the hourglass body type more typical of women, they will have a WHR lower than 1.0. A WHR close to 1.0 corresponds to a straight body type, which is more common among men and prepubescent children. Finally, if a person's waist is wider than their hips, they will have a WHR greater than 1.0 and very likely some form of belly. I haven't measured myself because mirrors are a thing, but I'm sure my WHR has always been above 1.0. Dr. Singh's early work showed that men, myself included, generally prefer women with a WHR of about 0.7, regardless of body size. Sarah's WHR has always been about 0.7, and the image of her pear-shaped figure perched on that stool in Tampa is forever seared into my memory. Women generally prefer

31 Our chats weren't always about psychology. At one point he asked about my summer plans, and I told him I was considering a trip to Europe or Australia. He recommended Europe, as Australia would have been a much more homogeneous experience. Later in life, when Sarah and I drove across Australia for a month, the phrase "Dr. Singh was right" became our unofficial motto. I loved every bit of Australia, but I can't think of a better single-word adjective for it than "homogeneous."

32 Dr. Singh was not the first to suggest the waist-to-hip ratio measurement, but his class was the first I had heard of it.

a WHR of about 0.95 in men, but lucky for me, there are other traits that can also make us attractive.

According to Dr. Singh, these preferences for body shape are not arbitrary; they have adaptive value. That is, ultimately they contribute to the survival of our species. Not coincidentally, the WHR judged most attractive for each sex is also associated with greater health and, more importantly for the propagation of the species, with fertility. The relationship to reproductive fitness is even more clear when you consider that WHR is generally the same for boys and girls before puberty, but once those hormones start deepening our voices and making our hair grow, our body shape changes and we enter the age of reproductive maturity. In adulthood, waist-to-hip ratio changes in women during pregnancy and menopause, two times in life when their reproductive potential is reduced. Hang on a minute—Sarah wants to take the mic. . .

> OK, ladies, so I know what you're thinking: *Does that mean that if I don't have Cardi B or J. Lo's booty, I'm not attractive or able to bear children?* That fear is what the beauty industry and plastic surgeons like to capitalize on, but we know the answer is no. There is truth in the old adage that beauty is in the eye of the beholder, with numerous physical and emotional characteristics attached to each person. Furthermore, while they're not always mutually exclusive in modern culture, there is a difference between beauty and hotness and the evolutionary sexual strategies that they tap into. First, because hotness, beauty, and attraction are related, albeit different, concepts that sexual mates and partners perceive for both short-term encounters and long-term

> relationships.[33] Second, and more importantly, even if you do have an ideal waist-to-hip ratio, even if you are in fact pregnant, that does not mean that the pelvic canal has the ability to open significantly farther than that of narrower-hipped female peers.[34]
>
> Speaking from personal experience, as someone who was told her entire postpubescent life that I have ideal childbearing hips and yet ironically found myself in a situation where child birthing was difficult, my doctor educated me that most women's pelvic canals are approximately the same size despite differences in their waist-to-hip ratio or bone structure. So perhaps all the WHR is really meaningful for is its ability to help us better identify who is male and who is female from a distance.

Yes, thanks, Sarah. See that? She's not just a collection of physically attractive features.

Because WHR, unlike some other physical traits, is visible from a distance, it allowed a primitive human to spot another primitive human across the savannah and instantly assess whether or not it was someone they would want to bone. Interpreting modern behavioral phenomena in terms of what they may have meant to early humans is the basis of evolutionary psychology, and Dr. Singh's class was my first exposure to that as well.

---

33 "The Science of Hotness vs. Beauty" (*The Joe Rogan Experience*, 2020), https://www.youtube.com/watch?v=PvQrFBOyDs0.

34 Jeanne Bovet, "Evolutionary Theories and Men's Preferences for Women's Waist-to-Hip Ratio: Which Hypotheses Remain? A Systematic Review" (*Frontiers in Psychology*, June 4, 2019), https://doi.org/10.3389/fpsyg.2019.01221.

A few more psychology classes, including an introduction to neuroscience, and I knew what I wanted to do with my life. My academic interest in eating and mating had its origin in Dr. Singh's class,[35] and when it came time for me to move on to graduate school, I wanted to focus my research on these subjects, with an evolutionary approach. Dr. Singh was even nice enough to help me with a letter of recommendation.

When I showed up at the University of New Orleans, I was eager to get into the brain and study eating and screwing. And I did exactly that. During my time in graduate school, I became intimately familiar with an area of the brain known as the hypothalamus.[36] The hypothalamus is located in the center of the brain and receives inputs from our senses and other areas of the brain, either directly or from its connections to the thalamus, the brain's relay station. In turn, it sends information out to other areas, either directly or by influencing the release of different hormones. It is an important structure that is involved in behaviors that help us live, such as regulating body temperature, the sleep-wake cycle, and eating; behaviors that help us survive, such as emotional responses like aggression and fear; and behaviors that help prolong our species, such as sexual behavior. If I was going to study eating and screwing, the hypothalamus was going to be my spot. Technically, I got to know the hypothalamus of the Long–Evans rat, one of many breeds bred specifically for laboratory research, but at this level, human and rat brains are pretty similar. Outside of the lab I also did a lot of eating and screwing, because this all went down in New Orleans.

---

35 My personal interest in eating and mating was already well established.

36 I am just introducing some of my experiences; I promise this is not about to turn into a textbook.

My first project[37] involved the ventromedial hypothalamus (VMH), a tiny part of an already tiny structure in the brain. The VMH is associated with satiety, signaling to the rest of the brain that we are full, and when it is damaged an individual loses the ability to say when. Shortly after having the VMH surgically removed, our subjects would start to gain weight and then get massive. They'd also get super aggressive, as the VMH also helped tell the brain when to stop biting the researchers. I never liked working with the VMH, mainly because I hated making hyperaggressive overweight animals, but I did find it interesting.

If the VMH tells us when to stop eating, the nearby lateral hypothalamus (LH) tells us when to start. When the LH is damaged, an individual will simply not eat even when given ample opportunity to do so. I used to think that if only we could either find a way to stimulate the VMH, tricking it into telling us we are full, or suppress the LH and prevent it from imparting a desire to eat in the first place, all my problems could be solved. Of course, the major obstacle to either of those becoming reality is that this form of brain surgery, at least the procedures we used in research, is not reversible, nor is it highly survivable. These are extremely small areas in the brain and hard to pinpoint with a high level of accuracy. Nonsurgical techniques would involve the use of chemical compounds, which would not be specific to these tiny areas of the brain. Looking back, I think it's funny that brain damage would seem more appealing than a healthy lifestyle of diet and exercise.

Damage to the VMH also interferes with sexual behavior, but my last bit of research using rats as subjects involved another

---

37 My first project after my initial surgical training.

part of the hypothalamus, the medial preoptic area (MPOA).[38] Stimulation of this area can induce erections in male rats and copulation if the male is in the presence of a receptive female.[39] The MPOA is seen as a structure pertaining to sexual motivation, or interest. I conducted a few studies on the MPOA, and one thing made clear throughout them all is that male rats will figure out a lot of mazes to gain access to a receptive female.[40] By the time I'd started this stage of my research, it had become apparent that I was developing an allergy to the animals, a common occupational hazard. Just being around them was bad enough, but studying them during sex (theirs) was too much. I had to move on.

I began designing experiments with humans, which meant no more brain manipulations. When I finished my doctorate, I returned to an idea I'd had in Dr. Singh's class about waist-to-hip ratio. I hypothesized that an individual's level of attractiveness (determined using WHR and other measures) and/or level of sexual motivation would influence the emphasis they place on attractiveness measures in others. Spoiler alert: it kinda does. This wasn't a groundbreaking piece of science,[41] but it helped get me where I am.

I have shared all of this to demonstrate that subjects related to body weight have been on my mind in an academic sense since

---

38 B.E. King, M.G. Packard, and G.M. Alexander, "Affective properties of intra-medial preoptic area injections of testosterone in male rats" (*Neuroscience Letters*, 1999).

39 Consent, unfortunately, has to be inferred with rats.

40 Just as I would eventually learn that a sexually motivated male human will drive from Los Angeles, California, to Boulder, Colorado.

41 My results were somewhat inconclusive. An artist blames his tools; I blame the obscure analytic method I used.

college, and, more importantly, to introduce some of the many ways food consumption and sexual behavior are related. Both behaviors are also pleasurable and rewarding, something I will elaborate on in a later section, and both are essential to the survival of our species.

Without going into too much detail, I also want to make sure I state that the hypothalamus is not the only area of the brain involved in producing these behaviors. Stick around and I'll discuss some of the other areas in a bit.

Eating and screwing are intricately linked behaviors. It was Sarah's fat distribution, measured by her optimal WHR, that caught my eye as she was perched on that stool in Tampa. Her shape[42] was an indication to the primitive areas of my brain that she was healthy and fertile, inspiring in me a desire to mate. The sight of her activated areas of my hypothalamus, increasing my motivation to interact with her. We were in a public space, a restaurant, and given the constraints this puts on our behavior, sex was not on the table.[43] However, eating food was (literally) on the table, and my hypothalamus also stimulated my desire to eat. Perhaps this served as a substitute for the other activity my brain desired, but it was the stated purpose of our meeting and much more socially acceptable. Sharing a pleasurable eating experience gave us an opportunity to bond over mutual interests, and eventually we got around to engaging in that other thing.

Another reason for sharing this was to describe some of the

---

42 Of course, she has many other qualities I find attractive. I am simplifying for the sake of this tie-in and would never reduce her or anyone else to a single attribute.

43 Pun very much intended. Besides, it was a counter.

mechanisms behind behaviors that many of us do not yet understand. My discussion of a few brain areas in no way presents an exhaustive assessment, but hopefully by reading a few details, you can see that our brains are not all thoughts and feelings. We aren't robots completely lacking in conscious awareness either, but a lot of our behavior is produced by structures outside of our conscious awareness. It may be unlikely that we will ever be able to take action on the mechanics of eating behavior, but it is important to understand that those mechanics exist. Understanding a bit about how the brain functions and why it functions that way can help us make some changes in our lives, as well as understand why change is so damn difficult.

Speaking of making changes, I am happy to report that when I stepped on the scale this morning, my weight was down another two pounds. I am resisting the urge to celebrate with ice cream.

CONSULTING THE EXPERT

Occupational Therapist Sarah Bollinger

A couple of years ago, I was asked to give the keynote address for the annual meeting of a group of occupational therapists. As you know, I identify as a comedian who also happens to have a doctorate in psychology, but they wanted me anyway. I began my talk by stating that I was not an occupational therapist but do share my life with one, and despite that, like most people, I am still not sure what they do. That got me a few laughs and helped to break the ice.

The part about not knowing was a joke, of course. The rest was true. Ever since a dinner date in Tampa, I have been sharing my life with an occupational therapist. I have already introduced Sarah Bollinger earlier in this book. She was also a certified life coach, and who better to discuss weight loss with than the coach sitting next to me?

Brian: First of all, what is an occupational therapist?

Sarah: An occupational therapist is a part of the health-care team that oftentimes falls under the umbrella of rehabilitation. My job is to help people become more independent in their everyday lives through occupation. What is occupation? It is literally anything you do to occupy your time. It encompasses a wide range of things such as basic health care, daily activities like self-care, and more complex ones like driving. We work with people of all ages and use a wide variety of techniques, including rehabilitation ones like strengthening and ones that adapt an environment or provide assistive tools. Overall, it has to do with looking at the person as an individual and a whole in order to bring more wellness and meaning to their life.

Brian: How often is weight loss a goal or an objective of the people you work with?

Sarah: It's not something that I would write as a goal when I do an evaluation and treatment plan for a patient, but it is definitely something that comes up in everyday treatment. Especially when people say things to me like, "I'm having this terrible back pain or knee pain," or "Is there anything else I could do to put myself in a better state of health?" Or when somebody is no longer in the acute stage, the stage immediately following an injury, and they are going home and want something more encompassing to wellness than the basics. I'll say, it would be great for your joints if we took some pressure off them. It comes up fairly often, even though it's not directly within our scope of practice. It falls under lifestyle redesign.

Brian: You are also a certified life coach. Can you tell me about that?

Sarah: I got into that through my own weight loss journey and then trying to use the skills I picked up to pay it forward and help others. I would say 99 percent, if not all, of my clients come to me for weight loss guidance. I let them know that the journey they'll need to take is not just about weight loss but more about health and wellness. Otherwise, they get too focused on the short term and the weight loss aspect only. Maintenance becomes more difficult and the real bigger picture of their life and sustained health falls to the wayside.

Brian: How do you go about coaching people to lose weight, and what sorts of advice do you give them?

Sarah: First and foremost, it starts with an interview, as in any health-care environment, just a little bit less formal, and getting realistic with them about why they want to lose weight. Why do they want to get healthy? The stronger the motivation, the more likely a person is going to be to achieve and maintain weight loss for the long term.

As for advice, the best time to start a new diet is when you are relaxed, not when you have anything big or stressful coming up. Find a realistic diet plan that you think you can actually stick to. Try to remember that you are not just trying to lose weight in the short term but retrain yourself to form healthier habits for the long term.

When I lost eighty pounds, I did a low-calorie, low-carb diet that consisted mostly of protein and vegetables. People often underestimate how much they are eating. When it comes to your exact caloric intake, that is something that you have to figure out based on your current activity level and lifestyle. Assistance of a professional and fitness trackers are helpful as well. People also tend to overestimate how much exercise they are doing.

Of course, we should always take advice with a grain of salt, but it is important to have a sense of accountability and the ability to confide in someone else. Whether it be a health coach, another health-care professional, or a very supportive friend who knows your goals, accountability is instrumental to weight loss and achieving our health goals.

Brian: I'm not one of your clients, but in helping me to lose weight, how difficult would you say I am?

Sarah: Well, you're a man [laughs] and you are my partner [laughs even harder], and nobody wants to listen to their family. Even when you have a family member who is a health-care provider, what could they possibly know? I have always found that my family members tended to ask me about health issues that I did not have expertise in, when they should have really been talking to their doctors. When I did have advice to offer, they didn't want to hear it much. And you are no exception to that. I had to fight you tooth and nail to go get sleep studies done! And to go to the doctor when I was pregnant with Alyssa! It was certainly a challenge.

Brian: What do you think my biggest mistakes are in regard to my health?

Sarah: I would say that as good as you are at calorie tracking, when it comes to those calories, you could stop and think more about what messages you are sending your brain with the types of food you are eating. When you look at it from a macro level, the calorie quantities are meaningful, but you also have to consider what's filling you up and what's providing nutrition to repair your body.

I would say that even though your CPAP [continuous positive airway pressure tool for sleep apnea] has helped you tremendously, you may still have some poor sleep habits in place. And get moving more, man! [laughs]

Brian: It's hard when you are writing a book.

Sarah: I know. It's always hard, even when you're not writing a book.

Brian: Have I been a difficult patient?

Sarah: I try not to look at you as my patient [laughs]. I don't think that's healthy for our relationship. Certainly, as a couple we could probably set some goals together to work on. Often for one person in a family to get healthy, the whole family has to get on board and get healthy. But yes, you've been difficult [laughs].

Brian: You have had your own ups and downs with body weight, and later in the book we'll share your story,[44] but you have a very active lifestyle. You are also a tango dancer and art model. How does body weight factor in to those activities?

Sarah: First of all, before all of those professions, I am just a person and I am a woman. I was raised in society like everybody else and I have a mirror in front of my face every morning like everyone else. I have one body and I feel how it moves and grooves or creaks. Body weight has a big part in how I feel in my mental health, my emotional health, and my overall well-being. Sometimes I am feeling more confident because I lost five pounds on the scale. That's sad because we shouldn't be assessed only by that stupid number we see, because that's not what makes up a person. But it certainly does influence how you're feeling sometimes.

As a health-care provider, I feel that it's important for me to

---

44 For those of you with a little less patience, feel free to skip ahead to the section labeled "Sarah's Struggle"—BUT WAIT! Please remember to come back when you are done!

be healthy, not only to perform my job duties but so I can be an example for my patients. I can say, "I know what it feels like to have those struggles" and "I know it is possible to accomplish these goals because I've done it before."

As a model, of course the overall idea in the industry is the thinner, the better [laughs]. I hate that mentality because it's simply not true. Thinner is not always healthier. There have been moments in my modeling when I have been thinner and I'm like, "Darn it, I lost all my boobies" or "I lost all my booty!" People like those curves too, because that's part of what makes you a woman. There are lots of different beauty standards. It's more important to me that I feel healthy and well.

Brian: As you know, my most recent attempt to lose weight is motivated by the fact that we have a daughter. I keep thinking to myself, *How do we raise a child without passing on our unhealthy tendencies?*

Sarah: I think it is like everything—we can model healthy behavior. Modeling desired behavior is more effective than simply telling her how to live, because you are leading by example. I think that will be a huge factor. The jobs of children are to learn and to grow, and they do so primarily through playing. Finding things that we enjoy together as a family will encourage our daughter. She's interested in different things, whether it's karate or swimming or other things that we cultivate. Let's get moving and try these things out together. Let's explore with healthy foods and maybe only treat ourselves to ice cream once in a while, and maybe when we are on the road let's see what healthy things we can find at the gas station. Let's make it a game. Children thrive on games.

Two Pounds of Fat

For as long as I can remember, I have made it a point to try any and all unusual foods that I encounter. I am no Andrew Zimmern, not even close, but whenever I have an opportunity to try something new, I usually take it. Nearly thirty years ago, while still in college, I was on a trip to New York City with a group of friends from Texas and saw jellyfish on a menu at a restaurant in Chinatown. I had no idea jellyfish was even edible and was immediately curious. When the waiter came around to ask me what I was interested in, of course I ordered the jellyfish. I remember him warning me, "People like you don't like jellyfish," which I perceived as a challenge. I told him I wanted to try it anyway, and he reluctantly took the order. A few minutes later he brought out all our food and placed a plate of what appeared to be jiggly brown noodles in front of me. I took one bite and instantly hated it. People like me don't like jellyfish.

Or maybe I need to try it again. I would be willing to give it another shot if I see it on another menu.

I've had shark fin soup, turtle soup, frog legs, snails, pig eyeballs, bull testicles,[45] chicken hearts, crawfish, horse meat, alligator and crocodile meat, kangaroo meat, and whatever sweetbreads[46] are. Clearly, I didn't gain all my weight by being a vegetarian. I

---

45 Is this list making you hungry yet?

46 I know what they are, but the first time I ordered them I really thought I was ordering a plate of *pan dulces* (Mexican pastries).

have even eaten tacos made with crickets, and somehow managed to keep them down. Not all of these foods are considered unusual by everyone, but they are certainly not typical of the American meatloaf-and-spaghetti diet I was raised eating. Occasionally I make videos with my family about eating exotic foods, making it even more fun to try something together. Earlier this year I learned that seal meat is legal to sell in Canada, and I became obsessed with the idea of eating a chunk of seal.[47] They say it is one of the most nutritious meats in the world, high in protein and low in fat, with more iron and calcium than most other meats. It isn't sold everywhere in Montreal, but I tracked some down and currently have two seal burgers in my freezer waiting for me to convince my family to make another video.

To my knowledge I have never eaten the brain of an animal. I am definitely not opposed, and I have seen them for sale in some markets, but I imagine it tasting like salty fat. Not that salt and fat aren't delicious as ingredients in pretty much every food, but I have never thought I wanted a whole plate of the parts of the steak I usually trim off. You may know that the brain is made up of individual cells called neurons, which conduct electricity, but you may not know that each of these is insulated from the others by supporting cells that are mostly made up of fat. The brain is full of fat, you fathead, and without salt the brain would be a useless lump of it. A neuron's ability to transmit electricity is facilitated by sodium and chloride ions, the charged particles created when salt is dissolved into water. The brain is about 60 percent fat, and with

47 I used to live a few blocks from Pier 39 in San Francisco, and sometimes the sound of the seals barking would echo all the way up to my apartment. Let's consider this meal payback for lost sleep.

those ions for flavor, I assume we get salty fat—although I have heard the taste of brain is similar to the taste of sweetbreads, so what do I know. Ask a zombie, or that woman in your office who brings in homemade *tamales de cabeza* every week.

This is a weird way to introduce another discussion on the brain, but given the overall theme of this book, I figure it is par for the course. Besides, when I get together with some of my neuroscientist friends, this is actually how we sometimes talk. In my book *The Laughing Cure*, I mentioned how police officers and people with similar occupations use a form of dark humor called gallows humor to deal with the stress of their work. It helps them cope with some of the terrible things they have to witness. The work of a neuroscientist is not nearly as stressful as the work of law enforcement, but let me tell you, we see some shit, man. Imagining the taste of brain hardly seems all that taboo, especially as human beings all over the planet regularly eat the stuff. You know what? This has motivated me to go eat some brains and make another video.[48]

The human brain weighs about three pounds on average, depending on how much obscure *Star Wars* trivia it contains. With about 60 percent of that being fat, I jokingly refer to it as two pounds of fat plus some other stuff. It is without a doubt the most important two pounds of fat in the entire body, regardless of what you paid for your butt augmentation. In the last section, I shared some insight into the roles that various nuclei of the hypothalamus have in mediating our eating and screwing.[49] However, those areas

48 I would too, if it weren't off the diet.

49 Two of the four Fs: fighting, fleeing, feeding, and fornicating. I could have used "eating and fucking," but then I'd risk my PG rating when this book comes out as a movie.

are only part of the system of brain that gets us wining, dining, and sixty-nining.

Earlier I described how in the beginning of my relationship I met Sarah for dinner in Tampa and that the detail I remember most vividly was the alluring sight of her fertility-signaling shape sitting on a stool as I arrived. Later I discussed how this visual cue was sufficient to get my hypothalamus revved up and motivate me to want to do a whole lot of hypothalamus-mediated things to her, but in the end my brain settled for some delicious Cuban food and conversation. The part of my brain that prevented me from going all animal style right there on the countertop was my prefrontal cortex, the home of my conscious mind.[50]

The prefrontal cortex is the part of the brain that lies directly behind the forehead and eye sockets. It is a small part of the brain overall, making up only about 10 percent of the brain volume,[51] but it is the home of everything we generally refer to as consciousness. I like to emphasize that it is the only part of our brain we are aware of. The brain is always active, doing all sorts of things important to living life, but most of that is outside of our awareness.[52] Our inner dialogue, decision-making, reminiscing on the past, or predicting future outcomes—all are behaviors that occur in the prefrontal cortex. It is the home of thought. You are using it right now as you read these words, and also as you say to yourself, "By the way, this book is the best book I have ever read." I'm glad you agree.

---

50 Her brain was definitely a factor too, but I am writing this from my brain's perspective.

51 And 60 percent of that is fat!

52 I suspect that the relatively small part of brain devoted to conscious thought is behind the myth that we only use a small portion of our brain. We use our entire brain, people! Stop perpetuating this ridiculous idea.

When I had that first encounter with Sarah and her 0.7 WHR, there were a lot of thoughts present in my conscious mind. I already had some idea of her personality from our previous interactions, I suspected there was mutual attraction, and I knew that the stated purpose of our meeting at a restaurant was to get to know each other better over dinner. I have also been raised in a society and have internalized many of the cultural norms. All of that information, stored in various parts of my brain, was accessible to my prefrontal cortex as I walked into that restaurant. Drawing from these sources, the prefrontal cortex has the ability to modify or override impulses from other areas of the brain. My thoughts, however much they may have been inspired by primal urges, were also the product of behavioral expectations and societal constraints. Just as I can find myself sexually attracted to someone and still act like a respectable human in her presence, I can also see a delicious-looking doughnut and resist the urge to toss it down my throat.

But as we all know, some urges are hard to say no to.

The prefrontal cortex is the part of our brain that makes conscious decisions, but it is not the only area of our brain that decides how we should behave. Sometimes we do things without conscious awareness. For example, Sarah, Alyssa, and I were at the dinner table last night. I would have started by stating that we were eating dinner last night, but really only two of us were eating. Sure, all three of us had a plate of food in front of us, but one of us has the brain of a five-year-old and is easily distracted. In the center of our table was an easel holding a freshly painted masterpiece by our daughter. The paint was not yet dry, something that Alyssa didn't seem to fully understand as she reached out to admire her work instead of eating her meal and got paint all over her hands. Sarah told her not to do that or she'd ruin the painting and make a mess. Then I also told her not to do it, but before I could even finish my sentence, she had her hands on the painting again. I asked her, "Why did you do that after Mommy and I both told you not to?"

If you're a parent, you will know exactly what her answer was: "I don't know," she said, and she was right. The decision to reach out and grab her painting was not made by the prefrontal cortex after evaluating her situation and analyzing the potential outcomes while taking her parents' requests into account. It was made by another area, the nucleus accumbens, without any conscious input. It was an impulse, an automatic behavior, a behavior commonly referred to as a habit. One job of the prefrontal cortex is to control impulses, a skill that a typical five-year-old brain has not quite mastered.

Before I go on, Sarah has something to add about controlling impulses:

> I'm sure that any parent who has been on an outing with their excited child or gone shopping in a place where novel objects are present has similar experiences with the need to redirect their child from touching something (or everything) on a shelf. It is not only normal curiosity but actually built into development and is a need from babyhood to first explore the world through eyes, then reaching, and then sticking objects in their mouths to learn how they feel and taste. Indeed, exploration of objects and environment through play is the very occupation of children and how they learn.

So how do we encourage exploration of environment within civilized and controlled social bounds? It starts with a simple knowledge of boundaries for safety within an understanding of the yes/no dichotomy, but yes/no is quite limited, not very open to understanding middle grounds, and can be quite paralyzing to a child who is by nature inquisitive.

Imagine you are a child (or a big kid at heart, because let's be realistic), and as you walk into a big, beautiful chocolate shop you are hit by an aroma of rich cocoa and surrounded by shelves, stands, and boxes of chocolates that have been hand-crafted, molded, and painted into stimulating shapes and colors, a sort of FAO Schwarz of chocolate.[53] Your eyes open wide, and you quickly run around to look at all the offerings. Your mouth is salivating, and naturally you want to grab and taste everything. You reach out for a wrapped chocolate teddy bear lollipop and *thwap*, your mother slaps your hand and sternly utters, "No!" From then on all it takes is a verbal "No . . . No . . . No," and most children get the point, but I doubt we really want to stop a child from exploring or experiencing. Hey now, though, let's be honest—did you bring your kid into this shop to tease or punish them? I'm sure that's not the case. Maybe the prices are not what you anticipated, but I'm pretty sure you just want them to exert a little self-control and not fall off the candy cliff. Impulse control is asking a lot from an adult but even more from a child who is innately wired to learn with

53 More from Sarah: "I am happy to report that such a chocolate shop exists in Dallas. It's a treasure and I won't tell you where it is, but I'll give you a real clue . . . it's a Secret! Also, thanks to the founder's son, who still works at the shop, any child who enters the store leaves with a free piece of chocolate (be sure to ask why). Now isn't that sweet?"

their primitive brain, a brain not yet fully developed and that requires the guidance of an adult.

When I was a young occupational therapist, I had a coworker who would watch me work with my patients and would often comment that one day I was going to be a great parent. I would ask why she was of that opinion, and she would say, "You really know how to push them out of the nest. Even more, you know how to teach them how to fly." The great parent part remains to be seen, as the show isn't over yet, but my approach to parenting has always been to openly guide exploration and encourage independence through meaningful experiences. With Alyssa, after her understanding of yes and no, we proceeded with "Be careful, it's fragile!" or "Be gentle," which are both quite effective at getting the point across quickly when children are learning. They understand fragile means something will break. In our family, that means OK to touch but explore with caution because your exploration could have irreparable consequences. We are quite the art enthusiasts, and I enjoy making pottery, so Alyssa learned early on how to handle fragile things. Still, to this day, I get a kick out of the nervous looks of museum volunteers or shop vendors as I let Alyssa carefully pick up a piece of pottery or a glass souvenir off a shelf.

Despite Alyssa's awareness, sometimes when we are out shopping, she will instinctively grab at something and say, "Mommy, let me see that!"

> I have to remind her, "OK, but look with your eyes, not with your hands," or, "OK, but remember, seeing is not touching." It takes practice and reinforcement. How many times have you impulsively grabbed a piece of candy off a countertop or coffee table just because it was there, without actually considering if you are hungry? Bargain stores like Dollar Tree (or Dollarama here in Montreal) thrive on this mechanism in your brain.

The nucleus accumbens is a relatively small but extremely important part of our brain. It is located near the center and receives input from several different areas including the prefrontal cortex as well as the amygdala, another area I have not yet mentioned. Put simply—because that is the only way I know how—the accumbens is the unconscious decision maker. It receives the same type of information that the prefrontal cortex gets and is capable of weighing out different options to decide on a course of action. The options it considers are simple behaviors that we have practiced so often throughout our lives that we can express them without any conscious input, like reaching for a painting at the dinner table. The nucleus accumbens uses a chemical called dopamine, which you may have heard of, especially in the context of understanding addiction. Dopamine is released when we engage in pleasurable behaviors, like reaching for a painting at the dinner table or consuming pleasurable substances. For this reason, many people refer to the nucleus accumbens as the pleasure center of the brain. This may be an easy way to think about it, but technically the nucleus accumbens has nothing to do with pleasure; it has to do with learning how to re-create pleasurable experiences (or avoid repeating painful ones). Dopamine activity in the nucleus accumbens is associated with a concept called reinforcement. The pleasure we feel comes from the activation of other systems.

Whenever our brain experiences something pleasurable or rewarding, cells in our nucleus accumbens start cranking out the dopamine. The more rewarding the experience, the more dopamine is produced. Therefore, the dopamine released can be viewed as a measure of how rewarding an experience is. Thanks to our body chemistry, some experiences—like having sex, using drugs, and eating doughnuts—are intrinsically more rewarding than others. Over time, we are bound to encounter repeated experiences, and if every time we engage in the same behavior we receive a reward, then that behavior is reinforced. Reinforcement is how the brain learns, and if we repeat an experience on a few occasions, each time with a positive result, the brain will remember to do it again.

Through reinforcement, the brain learns to repeat a behavior, and it also learns to anticipate the reward by associating it with frequently paired stimuli. These paired stimuli become predictors of future opportunities for reward and the triggers of cravings. You may have learned about Pavlov's experiments with dogs[54] or even trained your own. In Pavlov's version, food, a reward, was frequently paired with the ringing of a bell so that the dogs learned that when they heard the sound of the bell, food would be coming their way shortly. When the brain encounters one of its triggers in the environment, dopamine cells in the nucleus accumbens become active in anticipation. The greater the potential reward

54 Ivan Pavlov's work became the basis for what we now refer to as Classical Conditioning and has greatly influenced how we understand learned behaviors.

indicated by the trigger, the more active these cells become. This creates in us a sensation we may refer to as a craving, or a motivation. I prefer the word "urge" because it seems more general, but it is basically the same thing. In Pavlov's work, the dogs would salivate in response to hearing the bell, and if they could talk, they may have expressed an urge to eat.

My brain loves doughnuts. I know, I'm really expressing my individuality here, but it's true: my brain thinks doughnuts are very rewarding. As much as you can look at me and assume I am definitely no stranger to doughnuts, you have to appreciate that there was a time in my life when I'd never had one. Maybe I was a baby, although realistically I was probably a toddler. I don't remember that far back, nor have I asked my parents. Imagine my little toddler brain being given a doughnut for the first time: holding it in my hand, inspecting it, smelling it, and then putting a little in my mouth to see what all the fuss was about. And wow! That doughnut was amazing! I experienced pleasure, and my little toddler nucleus accumbens probably started producing buckets of dopamine as a result of that tasting. My toddler brain took note and thought, *This . . . this is something I need more of.* Over time I would have more, lots more, doughnuts, and with each positive experience my brain would get a reward, leading it to learn everything it could about how to re-create this doughnut pleasure. My brain would learn to associate the sight of doughnuts, the smell of the doughnuts, eventually even the word "doughnut," with the pleasure I received from eating them. These would eventually become the triggers of my doughnut craving. As I grew older, each positive experience with a doughnut would further strengthen the dopamine response in my nucleus accumbens. Eventually, I could find myself walking down the street, completely satiated after having a nice meal, and yet the smell of doughnuts coming from a nearby store would be enough to create an urge in me to go inside and buy, like, all the doughnuts. Like what happened earlier today. I'm kidding, but did you know that the word *beignerie* means "doughnut shop" in French? My brain now associates that word with the pleasure of eating a doughnut.

Speaking about motivation, let me go off script for a moment and state that very few things motivate us to action like food. Sure, a voluptuous woman shaking her booty in nothing but a thong can get me to do nearly anything (a fact that Sarah often uses to her advantage), but she could accomplish the same thing holding a well-cooked steak and she wouldn't even need to learn how to twerk. The lure of food, good food, can be powerful.

As I mentioned in the very beginning of this book, literally the second paragraph, in college I worked as a counselor at a summer camp. Specifically, I worked with ten-year-old boys. Campers were not allowed to bring any food with them, and candy was considered contraband. Each group of campers spent about two weeks with us before going home, and for most of that time we were able to encourage good behavior and cooperation from the kids by threatening to take away activities they enjoyed, like swimming or playing games. You know, if you don't get your cabin clean, we are going to have to cancel our time at the lake! On the last day of their encampment, we needed each kid to help prepare the camp for the next group, but since they were leaving, the campers knew they had nothing to lose and would always become very difficult to wrangle. That's when I would break out a box I kept hidden under my bunk. With all the kids gathered around, I would open it and ask them what was inside.

"That's candy!" they would shout with excitement.

"No," I'd correct them, "that's motivation." I started this practice during my second encampment, and from that point forward, the chores always got done.

I still remember one of the kids coming up to me and asking, "Mr. Brian, can I please have my motivation now?"

So back to how the brain makes unconscious decisions. Throughout my life, my brain has learned that millions of different behaviors and experiences are potentially rewarding. My brain not only likes eating doughnuts, but it has learned to enjoy healthier options like carrots and cauliflower as well. Um, yummy. Each option inspires the associated cells in my nucleus accumbens to produce dopamine at different rates. If my brain simultaneously recognizes more than one opportunity for reward at the same time, whichever option is associated with greater dopamine activity is the one the nucleus accumbens is going to pick. For example, imagine that I find myself at a party and the host has put out a snack table with an assortment of doughnuts and a plate of fresh veggies[55]—you can probably guess which snacks I will start to crave. I may have every intention of sticking to my diet, but if my conscious mind is busy having a conversation with someone or otherwise distracted so that I am not paying close attention to my behavior, I'm going to grab a doughnut. No conscious thought

55 Because at my age, all imaginary parties include snack tables.

needed. It is all too easy to absentmindedly act out of habit, making weight loss a real challenge.

Estimates differ, but most researchers agree that the majority of all of our behavior is unconsciously motivated. Very little of what we do is the result of rational decision-making. When my daughter said she didn't know why she grabbed the painting, she was speaking the truth. Just like when I popped into the beignerie on my way home earlier. Why did I do that if I am trying to lose weight and write a book about weight loss? I don't know.

It's all in that two pounds of fat.

In my discussion of reinforcement, I have focused on experiences that are pleasurable, or rewarding. This is referred to as positive reinforcement, and as I have described, it results in increasing the likelihood of repeating a behavior. It is important to recognize that reward is not the only form of reinforcement; we also learn to repeat behaviors that relieve pain or discomfort. This is referred to as negative reinforcement. My go-to example for this is usually taking aspirin for a headache, but because I seem to be in a doughnut state of mind right now, I'll continue along those lines. Let's imagine I suffer from hypoglycemia and have a headache, feel dizzy, and am having difficulty concentrating. Recognizing these as symptoms of low blood sugar, I look around for something sweet and see a box of doughnuts from a nearby shop conveniently placed within reach. Without questioning how or why these doughnuts happened to find their way into my office, I reach for one and take a bite. Moments later I start to experience relief from my discomfort, and cells in my nucleus accumbens are squirting out dopamine. I did a thing, and as a result I experienced relief from my pain. This is negative reinforcement. The next time I feel the onset of symptoms, I will have an increased likelihood to grab a doughnut. In this case, doughnuts are both offering me pleasure and helping to relieve my symptoms, which increases the likelihood of repetition even more.

Learning is multifaceted. There are also experiences that decrease the likelihood of repetition. These are referred to as punishment. For example, imagine I bite into a doughnut and it tastes absolutely horrendous, causing me to spit it out in disgust. If that was my experience from the beginning, my little toddler brain would have never picked up another doughnut again. Similarly, if, after already developing a taste for them, I find myself repulsed every time I attempt to enjoy another, eventually my nucleus accumbens would show lower and lower levels of dopamine activity until it gets so low that some other option becomes better in comparison. Therefore, the behavior of eating doughnuts would be completely extinguished.

Hypothetically, let's imagine that unrestrained doughnut consumption is the sole reason for my excess weight gain. If I want to lose weight by modifying my caloric intake, I would either have to convince my brain that despite years of contradictory experiences, eating doughnuts provides neither pleasure nor relief from low blood sugar, or I would have to somehow convince my brain that doughnuts are repulsive. Yeah, good luck with that. This is part of the reason why losing weight is so difficult. And that's just one type of food!

I have always assumed that I am working with a fully functioning, relatively healthy brain. I may not be, as I have never had my brain scanned, and it has been a while since my last IQ test. Perhaps years of unhealthy living have permanently affected my brain in some unknown way, but with no evidence to the contrary, I like to think that the two pounds of fat living in my skull have been safely insulated from the misdeeds of my other organs.[56] My brain works, and it seems to work really well. I have also been overweight my entire life. The crazy thing is, I have always known how to lose weight *and* I have always had the desire to do so, *and yet* my supposedly healthy functioning brain has been unable to accomplish this goal.

This is a point that I usually make to emphasize how hard it is to change our behavior. I know smart, successful people who have lost everything because their brain kept choosing to use drugs and alcohol. I know health-care professionals who, despite their extensive knowledge, are heavy smokers, and many of them also deal with various levels of obesity. The adult brain has a capacity to support change, but realistically speaking, it is highly unlikely to do so. Our brains are like your deadbeat ex-boyfriend begging to get you back: "Come on, baby; I can change. Just give me another chance!" I think we all know this. This isn't news. Nearly every person reading this paragraph has probably attempted some form of behavioral change and been unsuccessful. And regarding your ex-boyfriend, please don't fall for that crap again, Judy. You are better than that.

I used to make this point to help explain why so many of us maintain unhealthy behaviors despite knowing better and having a desire to change. In some ways it helped me to resolve the obvious incongruence of being a big fat guy and teaching people

56 Give it up for the blood-brain barrier, ladies and gentlemen!

about behavior change. However, after sharing this message for so long, it began to weigh[57] on me. Perhaps setting a positive example would send a message more important than explaining why change is so hard.

Change is extremely hard, and that is the reason why, as I write this, I still have a lot of extra weight to lose. The struggle is real, and all I can do, all any of us can do, is do what we can as best as we can. Change won't happen overnight, and the short-term payoffs are minimal, but we absolutely can and do change.

FAT TALES

Time to Bring the Doughnuts

In order for the conscious mind to exert control over our tendency to engage in automatic responses, it has to be aware of what we are doing and paying attention. And yet, even if both of those things are occurring, even if we are fully paying attention and very much aware of our behavior, our decision-making can be more influenced by the urges of the nucleus accumbens than the rational thinking of the prefrontal cortex.

That is because, relative to the nucleus accumbens, the prefrontal cortex is really slow. You may recall that the nucleus

57 Pun very much intended.

accumbens makes a decision by comparing the relative activity of dopamine cells. That is a very simple decision to make. It is basic math to show that this quantity is greater than this quantity. The nucleus accumbens makes decisions so quickly that the response is almost automatic. As you are probably aware, your conscious mind, which lives in the prefrontal cortex, is capable of factoring a whole lot of information into decision-making, and very often it does exactly that. However, all those extra analyses that we conduct slow down the decision-making process. Sometimes our conscious mind is too slow to influence the decisions made by our unconscious.

When I first started touring as a public speaker, I was still living in San Francisco and would often share the following story as an example.

> I live in San Francisco, California, and I absolutely love it. However, like in any city there are going to be things you like about it and things that you don't like. One of the things I don't like about San Francisco is that there are no good doughnut shops. None.[58] If you've ever been out there, I know you didn't go for the doughnuts. We don't have any good doughnut shops. Now, in my opinion, the greatest doughnuts in the world are the ones made by Krispy Kreme. Krispy Kreme is like crack. Seriously, they are that good. If you haven't tried them, don't! I definitely do not advocate anyone start that habit. But nonetheless they are really good and I like them. When I first moved to San Francisco, I was disappointed to find out there were no Krispy Kremes in the

58 Keep in mind, this was a while ago and things may have changed.

city, or decent doughnuts in general. And then I learned that the closest Krispy Kreme was a few miles south of the city on Highway 280. Because I was new to the area, I did not have a lot of experience driving down that highway. So the first few times I drove that way, it was for the sole purpose of getting doughnuts. Then, because the only times I had driven down that road were to get Krispy Kreme, I accidentally trained my brain to associate doughnuts with driving down Highway 280. Now the highway triggers a craving, and every time I drive down that way, whatever the reason may be, I can't help thinking to myself, *Hey, I can get Krispy Kreme!* It's an idea that pops into my head as a response to driving down 280.

One day not too long ago, I was driving down that way and the thought popped into my head about doughnuts and that in turn led to a full prefrontal analytic dialogue. I'm going to anthropomorphize a bit and describe my thought process like this: First, a part of my conscious mind said, "Sure, we can get Krispy Kreme; it's not like we drive down here very often," to which another part of my conscious mind chimed in, saying, "Well, we are trying to make better decisions, healthier decisions, and you know doughnuts aren't really a good option. Let's skip the doughnuts." Then, the original part of my conscious mind answered back and said, "Well, we could just get one. There's no harm in getting one doughnut, right?"

To which the other part of my conscious mind answered back and said, "OK, you know that's impossible. You can't get one doughnut. You know you are going to get the special doughnut, a couple of regular glazed, and before you know it, you'll realize that it would be cheaper to get a dozen. You know damn well that you are going to end up with a car full of doughnuts!"

And, of course, the other part of my conscious mind answered back, "Yeah, you're right about that. But you know, they *do* have good coffee. We were going to stop for coffee anyway—let's get coffee there!"

Finally, the other part of my conscious mind answered back and said, "OK, quit trying to trick me. You know we are not just going to get coffee if we stop."

So that's actually a pretty accurate description of my thought process that day, but what I am getting at is there was an active debate going on in my prefrontal cortex about whether or not I should pursue this option. And that debate ended when I realized I'd parked my car in the Krispy Kreme parking lot.

I know.

I had no conscious awareness of pulling off the highway and driving into their parking lot. It is as if—and I am going to anthropomorphize again here—my nucleus accumbens said, "OK, you guys can debate all you want. This represents an opportunity for a tremendous amount of reward based on past experiences, and we are doing it." My unconscious nucleus accumbens made the decision without conscious input, while my conscious mind was actively thinking about it.

This happens all the time. Very often our behavior is the product of unconscious motivations that are sometimes contrary to what our stated intentions may be. We do things all the time because our prefrontal cortex is too slow to influence the decision.

I'll end this story by sharing that I caught myself in the last minute. I started to get out of the car and realized, *What am I doing here? I don't want doughnuts!* I got back in the car and left. I am proud to say that I didn't get any doughnuts that day.

I got them the next day. And they were delicious.

I can't remember how many times I told a version of that story, but I know it always went over well. Sarah even claims that I told it at the first seminar she attended with me, and she's probably right, because her memory for such things is better than mine and she's going to read this. It became something that I was known for, the doughnut story. I would get emails from people who related to it or shared it with others, and all of that is awesome.

The craziest thing was that at some point, without irony, people started bringing me doughnuts.[59] On a number of occasions people would bring me some from a nearby Krispy Kreme or whatever local doughnut shop they thought I should try. I am familiar with famous comedians with signature bits like Jim Gaffigan, whose Hot Pockets routine has encouraged lots of fans to gift him with Hot Pockets, but I never expected my story to be one of

59 Or showing me recent pictures of doughnuts on their phone, which is how I initially bonded with my friend Denise in Oregon.

those bits. For about the first year, each time it happened, I would post a photo of me with the doughnuts to social media, something that may have further fueled the trend. Had I known this would happen, I would have made the story about twenty-dollar bills or something more useful. Still, each time I was very appreciative and ate all the doughnuts. I decided to quit telling that story for my own health.

Sorry, but the Bear Is Back

There is another part of those two pounds of fat worth mentioning, an area called the amygdala. The amygdala is a bilateral, almond-shaped structure that lies within close proximity of the hypothalamus, nucleus accumbens, and prefrontal cortex. By location alone you can probably guess that it is related to eating and screwing, and you would be right with that guess. Congratulations, you have amazing powers of deduction. Also, you've been paying attention to the context.

The amygdala's primary role is to detect threat. The word "primary" may be a bit of a judgment call on my part, but given how important being able to quickly identify threats in our environment is to our overall survival, I give it the top spot on the list. It is common to discuss the amygdala as the emotional center of the brain, and it has a role in our affective experience, but a lot of that is related to threat detection as well. Every time we encounter something in the world, the first thing our brain has to do is quickly answer the question "Is that thing going to kill me?" with a simple yes or no. The amygdala does this fast, really fast, and often before the prefrontal cortex has an opportunity to speak up.

When the amygdala decides that a stimulus is threatening, it sends a signal to other parts of our brain that activate our autonomic nervous system. This system is a network of nerves that extend from the brain down the length of the spinal cord and produce changes in a whole bunch of bodily organs. Our pupils will dilate, our heart rate will increase, our stomach will get all knotty, we will perspire, our bladder will relax, stuff like that. You may recognize these changes as part of our stress response. That's because stress is our brain's reaction to a perception of threat. The amygdala is so quick to assess threat that many of the physiological changes that take place in the body as a response will happen before we have conscious awareness of whatever we have encountered.

In my previous book, *The Art of Taking It Easy*, I used my favorite example of a hypothetical threat: being attacked by a big grizzly bear. My publisher even chose an image of a scary-looking bear for the cover, which is why my five-year-old daughter prefers my first book.[60] I say this is my favorite example not because I have some morbid fascination with bear attacks, or a highly specific kink, but because it is grounded in reality. I live in North America, a continent that human beings share with bears. I should note that on many occasions, I have encountered bears in the wild, but

60 When you are learning how to read, it's OK to judge a book by its cover.

I have never actually felt threatened by them. Most of the time they have either ignored me or seemed to feel threatened by my presence, but nonetheless I know that they can, and sometimes do, attack. I've used other examples, both real and fictional animals, but none seem to work for me like imagining a giant angry bear standing up on its hind legs and threatening to maul me to shreds. In addition, I think the example is relatable. Most of us would agree that if we somehow found ourselves in that situation, it would be quite stressful. I know I'd probably relax my bladder pretty damn quick. Also, and this is really important to me, bear attacks are extremely rare, so hopefully nobody reading this is suddenly being flooded with bad memories. I suppose there are other realistic yet extremely rare examples of potential threats in the world, but this is going to be brief, so I think I'll stick with the bear attack.

So imagine seeing a bear in the distance in obvious attack mode. Our sense organs bring information about the bear into our brain as we see it, smell it, and hear it. That information is processed and sent to the amygdala, which determines it to be a threat and activates the autonomic nervous system, resulting in some physiological changes taking place in the body. Those changes will take place prior to our prefrontal cortex having conscious awareness of the situation. It is a split second, but imagine that we suddenly realize there is a bear attacking us and our body has already responded by increasing our heart rate, tightening our stomach, and so on. Our prefrontal cortex will integrate this information in the thoughts we think, the emotions we feel, and the behaviors we engage. It is as if the prefrontal cortex says, "OK, there is a bear present. My heart is beating really fast and my stomach feels tense. Therefore, I must be afraid."

Of course, this is an extremely simplified description of how this works, but it's not wrong. Our emotions are based on multiple inputs, and if our amygdala perceives a threat, that is likely to lead us to feel some sort of stress-based emotion. These are usually negative, such as fear, anger, and sadness, but they can also be positive, such as excitement, depending on the stimulus and interpretation. If our amygdala perceives the situation as nonthreatening, well then that opens up a whole other set of possible emotions, depending again on the interpretation. So the amygdala detects threat and that influences our emotions. This is why the amygdala is commonly referred to as the emotional center of the brain. We don't feel emotions in our amygdala, but its activity contributes to them a great deal.

I can't speak for everyone, but emotions are an important part of my eating.

Unless it is jellyfish, consuming food is pleasurable. Whenever I am in a good mood, treating myself to a nice meal or an indulgent snack is icing on the proverbial cake.[61] Oh man, now I want cake. This isn't strange, is it? We celebrate everything with food. Is it your birthday? Let's hit an all-you-can-eat Brazilian churrascaria! And then get cake. Did you get a promotion? I know the perfect place we should go out to eat to celebrate! Most of our holidays are celebrated with food. We go crazy for candy on Halloween, Valentine's Day, and Easter and buy holiday-themed candy for half price on the days after Halloween, Valentine's Day,

---

61 Unless it is literal cake.

and Easter. Is there any other way to celebrate Mother's Day then to take her to brunch? Is it even the Fourth of July without a barbeque? Graduating? Let's eat. Getting married? Let's eat. Getting divorced? Let's eat. You say your STD test came back negative? Let's have sex. And then eat.

The amygdala's role in our desire to eat should be obvious, as eating has a huge emotional component. However, as I mentioned, the primary role of the amygdala is to detect threat, so how does stress play into our appetite?

Once again, imagine you are being attacked by a giant, ferocious bear. It clearly intends to do you harm, and your brain has correctly identified it as a threat. You have activated the autonomic nervous system, and an entire set of changes have taken place in the body. Those changes are designed to help you perform some action, whatever it may be, that will hopefully help you survive the impending bear attack. It is highly likely that your behavior is going to fall into one of two categories: fight or flight. That is, you are either going to do something aggressive, like prepare to defend yourself (or even attack), or you are going to try to remove yourself from the situation, like run or hide. Fight or flight represents our two basic responses to anything threatening.

I love the phrase "fight or flight." It characterizes the behavioral responses to stress so well, and so concisely, and is a beautiful combination of words like we almost never see in science. Fight and flight rhyme, they are single syllable words, and they both start with F. It is a work of art, poetry, which is why it annoys me so much when people want to ruin that perfect phrase by adding a third or fourth option. Why mess with perfection? Especially when the entire point is to simplify behaviors into a small number of categories. The most common way people screw up the phrase "fight or flight" is by adding the word "freeze," which is . . . whatever. At least it starts with F and is only one syllable. Anyway, let me get back to that bear attack.

Actions require energy, and if you are being attacked by a bear, your brain wants to make sure everything that you do helps to increase your chance of survival. Anything that you do that is not directly related to either fighting or fleeing is wasted energy and might get you killed. For example, in the face of that charging bear, it is probably not a good idea to suddenly have the urge to eat. Although bears can be tasty.

By the way, I just remembered that I have also eaten bear meat. I didn't think of it earlier because it was from my friend's hunting trip in Colorado, not store-bought. Also, it was made into a sausage, and anything made into sausage loses its original appearance. It's not like I got to take a bite out of a paw. Anyway, sorry for the interruption.

If you are being attacked by a bear, one of the last things you want to do is stop to make a sandwich. Obviously, we need energy to fight or flee, and our food is where our energy comes from, but you aren't going to be able to eat, process that food, and make it available to the cells that need it in time to use it to survive the bear attack. It would make no sense to see that bear and say, "Oh, I should probably carb up!" That's not how things work. The act of eating also uses a lot of energy, which is energy that could have been put to better use running from or defending ourselves against the bear.

For this reason, when our amygdala perceives a threat in our environment, it sends a signal to the hypothalamus, which in turn signals the release of a hormone called cortisol into our blood. We commonly refer to cortisol as the stress hormone, and it has a number of additional effects on the body, including loss of appetite. We don't feel like eating when we are under stress, which is a good thing if that stress is being caused by an actual threat to our continued existence. The loss of appetite is real, despite the fact that during stress some of us gain weight, and there are many people who lose a lot under chronic stress. But before you go thinking, "Ah, the stress diet! That's the one I haven't tried yet!" keep in mind that this is a terrible way to lose weight.

Most of us have experienced a stress-related loss of appetite, at least for the short term. On my last tour, a guy came up to me and told me about a busy week he had at work. He said that there was one day in particular that was so demanding that he forgot to eat. After learning about appetite suppression during stress, he realized that it wasn't that he forgot to eat but that his brain never acknowledged that he was hungry. That has happened to me a lot too, and I am sure you can relate as well. I asked him what happened when he finished his work that day, and he replied, "Oh, man, I ate so much!" We won't eat when we are being attacked by a bear, but as soon as that bear is gone, let's hit the buffet.

Another reason it is probably not a good idea to eat when we are being attacked is the act of eating diverts our attention and makes us vulnerable. There is a popular movie trope used to show how badass or insane a character is by having them calmly eat a meal during circumstances that would make most of us very uncomfortable. Most mob movies have such a scene. My favorites are in *Goodfellas*:[62] the dinner scene where Tommy, played by Joe Pesci, asks Henry, played by Ray Liotta, "How am I funny?" and the scene when they sit down to a nice meal with Tommy's mother and joke about the dead man in their trunk. This trope is also used to show how desensitized coroners or morticians can become and seems so common that almost every scene that takes place in a morgue includes someone nonchalantly chomping down on food. I don't personally know any morticians, but I would be surprised if they chose to rest their lunch on a cadaver.[63] It is a powerful image that works as a shortcut to our brain telling us that this person does not feel threatened.

Unbothered eating is a behavioral display of confidence. To this day, I still remember one of the executives from the very first company I worked for after college. He had this peculiar practice of eating lunch alone in our cafeteria with his back facing the entire room of people. That simple posture conveyed to everyone that he knew he had nothing to worry about. Hell, I have nothing to worry about, and I still prefer to eat with my back to a wall in my own home.

If stress knocks out our appetite, why then do so many people gain weight when they are stressed? There is actually a simple reason for this, and it is the same reason people gain weight in general. Human beings are really good at eating when they are not

---

62 Still one of my absolute favorite movies ever.

63 I asked my social network, and as I suspected, my very small sample of respondents all reported that they would never do this and never saw anyone they worked with doing it. Although my friend and fellow comedian Minda Kistner added, "After I sew up an autopsy, the craving for ribs is strong. All of us are like that."

hungry. We are masters of that particular skill, better by far than any other species.

There are a lot of reasons human beings gain weight, and I am sure that they all contribute to the obesity epidemic. A lot of people discuss how portion sizes and/or caloric density have increased over time, and those no doubt factor in. Many place the blame on the incredible availability of food. We—at least those of us with sufficient means living in developed nations—are surrounded by an abundance and variety of food. In the United States, and Canada to some degree,[64] I can more or less have whatever I want whenever I want it. The presence of abundant calories has definitely contributed to my weight gain, as I don't have to look too far back to remember the last time I raided the fridge for a midnight snack (it was yesterday). However, we aren't the only species to live with such abundance. Before I met Sarah, I had a dog named Luna (I used to mention her often in my seminars, which is probably why Sarah recalled writing down her name the first time she saw me), and Luna lived with an abundant food source as well. For twenty-four hours a day, seven days a week, I made sure her food dish was fully stocked. She could eat as much as she wanted whenever she wanted, and yet she never ate more than she needed. She would eat when she was hungry and stop eating when she had enough. I'm not denying that some domesticated animals become obese in our society, but unless people's homes are filled with fat dogs and cats that never go outside,[65] it is far less frequent than with us humans.

---

64 There are a few things I have learned I cannot get in Canada, and a few things I cannot get when I am back in the States.

65 That seems strangely possible now that I phrase it that way.

A big reason why we pack on the pounds is that we have learned how to eat when we are not hungry. There are so many reasons to eat that have nothing to do with hunger. For me, on my way to becoming a four-hundred-pound man of mass (guy of girth?) I have eaten a lot, and I bet actual hunger factored into a small percentage of that. Sure, I eat when I am hungry, but I also eat out of boredom. I eat to be social. I eat to avoid wasting food or money (finish your plate!). Speaking of money, after voluntarily spending a long period of my life in institutionalized poverty, otherwise known as college, I developed a particularly unhealthy habit of never refusing free food, so if someone else is buying, I'm usually eating, regardless of my hunger level.

I remember hearing some advice on the radio last holiday season in Texas. The on-air personality read what she thought was a good trick to help manage calories: eat a healthy snack before you go to the Christmas party if you think that you might overdo it on the sweets. Yeah, because hunger is why people overdo it on sweets at parties. Spoken like someone who doesn't understand what "overdoing it" means. I don't care how much tofu I have in my gut, there is always room for Christmas cookies and chocolate. The best way to avoid the urge to eat at a party is not to go; the second best way is to stay the hell away from the snack table.

I have eaten things on a dare. I have eaten things to win bets. One of the dumbest reasons I eat has got to be so that I don't have to put a half-empty container back in the fridge or cupboard. I used to joke that I didn't understand the purpose of a chip clip. I mean, who can't finish a bag of chips? Or how some "king-sized" candy bars are actually split into two smaller candy bars and have text on the package that reads something like "Enjoy half now, save half for later!" I have never saved half for later. How can you leave an unfinished candy bar?

By far I think the stupidest reason I ever ate something was for attention. This isn't true of everyone, but most comedians are basically attention whores. I used to say that comedians were wannabe rock stars who never learned to play an instrument. If I could trade places with any member of even a mediocre band with a steady gig schedule, I probably would. Even the bass player. Although I was slow to adopt it, I became a comedian in the era of social media. I saw a few comics rise in popularity thanks to Myspace,[66] which was already starting to die before I ever stepped on a stage. Facebook and Twitter were rising, and I embraced both, although I enjoyed Facebook more in the early days. Unlike Facebook, Twitter restricted all posts to 140 characters, and for some reason I had a hard time being funny using anything less than 150. I never developed much of a following on Twitter, other than fake accounts, and on Facebook I still struggle to call myself a "micro-influencer." I was a late adopter when Instagram became popular, despite also being a prolific photographer (another thing Sarah noted when she first attended my seminar), but eventually I started to see the value. My first few posts were of food, especially the strange or excessive meals I would find on the road. Surprisingly, these posts were popular, and every like or comment hit my brain with enough shots of dopamine to encourage me to keep filling my feed with pictures of food.

When I started touring, there was a show on the Travel Channel that caught my attention called *Man v. Food*. It starred

66 Does Dane Cook ring a bell?

actor Adam Richman and happened to film episodes in many of the cities I was scheduled to visit. If you are unfamiliar with the show, each episode would take Adam to a different city to participate in some local food challenge such as the famous seventy-two-ounce steak at the Big Texan Steak Ranch in Amarillo, which is free if you can eat it in an hour.[67] In preparation for the main event, he would visit a few other spots in each city with various high-calorie offerings. His show become a sort of travel guide for me at a time when posting food pictures to social media was still common. I never did any of the food challenges, but I ate plenty of oversized meals that received "Was that the place from *Man v. Food*?" comments on social media. Again, this was probably the stupidest reason I ever ate.

Eventually I found myself in Denali, Alaska, and posted a photo of a Bloody Mary with an unusually large garnish of meats and cheeses. It got a lot of attention.[68] Before then I had enjoyed an occasional bloody, but at that point I started seeking them out. For a few years, loaded Bloody Marys garnished with everything from hamburgers to fried chickens were Instagram gold, and as I toured the country, I collected photos of all that I could. I became more known for my consumption of tomato-based cocktails than for my jokes, and I was invited to judge Bloody Mary festivals all over the country. I got to know bartenders, restaurant owners, other writers, and all sorts of bloody aficionados in the process. I wrote my own Bloody Mary travel guide,[69] which I sold at events,

---

67 I haven't attempted this yet, but part of me still kind of wants to.

68 At least compared to most of my other posts at that time.

69 Due to the pandemic, and the tumultuous nature of the restaurant industry, I suspect a number of the places listed in my guide may be closed. However, if you are interested in checking it out, it's *A Field Guide to the North American Bloody Mary* (independently published, 2018).

and even attempted to pitch a Bloody Mary–themed TV show. Thankfully, a lot of that buzz eventually died down and I never got a chance to become the Bloody Mary version of Adam Richman. In his *Man v. Food* days, Adam was not a very big guy, but he was always chubby, and publicly he has stated that starring on the show took its toll on him. After four seasons, he moved on and has since gotten into really good shape. Occasionally I still enjoy a good Bloody Mary, but I no longer seek them out.

So how do we learn to eat when we are not hungry? I had always assumed this was something I didn't have to learn, as I have no recollection of acquiring the skill. However, my thoughts on that subject changed last year during a conversation I had with my daughter, Alyssa. The conversation took place at a hotel one morning when Sarah and I asked her to have some breakfast before we started our day. She said she wasn't hungry, initiating a conversation that I suspect most parents have with their children, and we told her that we understood she wasn't hungry but that it was important she ate something anyway because later on, while we were working, she would not have the opportunity. We all know how complicated life can get. As adults, most of us have times during the day we have designated for meals, and we understand the need to eat when we have the chance, but my four-year-old didn't have a job with work she needed to schedule around. Her body wasn't trained to get hungry and need refueling around lunchtime. Just as the words left my mouth, I had a sudden realization that this could be the start of teaching her to eat when she is not hungry, so I quickly reversed my position. Sarah and I discussed it, and we decided that rather than try to force Alyssa's appetite to conform to our schedule, we would rather her eat only when she is hungry for as long as she can. One of the best things I can do for my daughter is help her avoid developing the same bad habits I continue to struggle with.

Thankfully, when it comes to raising my daughter, I have Sarah's help. She adds:

> Although we are certainly built with survival in mind and our brain is built to seek out sweet, salty, and fatty foods, factors of environment and exposure and learned behaviors also certainly play a role. Our daughter, Alyssa, was never exposed to sweet foods until we celebrated her first birthday. She got such a kick out of being given permission to play with her food, and watching her smash up and squish her cheesecake, all the while giggling nonstop, was adorable.[70] She didn't actually eat much cake that day, but the moment she got some of the whipped cream in her mouth, her face lit up and you could almost see the receptors in her brain firing, as if a light switch had been flipped. This is your brain on sweet! We quickly asked the waiter to bring some more whipped cream. To this day, she will often ask for a bowl full of whipped cream with cinnamon! Yum! Yet, we were surprised how many times she had to try chocolate before she started enjoying it. I am surprised that she still doesn't like foods like fruit snacks or maple syrup because they are too sweet.

---

70 Sarah goes on, "By the way, if you ever decide to let your child smash a birthday cake, I highly recommend doing so at a restaurant. The table and floor cleanup are so much easier. Tip your server well."

> While I certainly want my child to enjoy the good life, and fatty foods like peanut butter and Goo Goo Clusters have historically played their roles in survival, I don't push any unhealthy food too much. I have no doubt that she will develop lots of other equally adaptive food preferences in their place. Once upon a time, though, she loved to eat broccoli, spinach, pickles, lemons, and an assortment of other healthy foods. They say that taste buds change over time, but somewhere between babyhood and becoming a kid, those receptors have certainly diminished. I have no doubt that the frequent portrayal of kids who despise vegetables in cartoons and movies is partly responsible. Negotiating at the dinner table is commonplace, but we keep exposing her anyway in hopes that broccoli will eventually stick again like chocolate (a parent can hope, right?). In the meantime, you can't celebrate everything with ice cream, a little balance is in order, and three more bites of broccoli before you can be dismissed.

We are capable of eating when we are not hungry, and therefore many of us gain weight despite the appetite suppression brought on by stress. That is definitely part of the problem. Another factor is something I mentioned earlier, that eating is pleasurable. It feels good to consume food, and some foods, particularly those high in carbohydrates, actually have mood-elevating properties. This makes sense. Sugar is a source of energy, and having a pleasant response to consuming sugar helps ensure that we will continue to eat it. Stress can make us feel bad, and eating foods rich in carbohydrates can make us feel better, even if it is only temporary relief. This is why comfort foods are a thing. Stress eating is a real phenomenon. Studies have shown that the amygdala has a role in stress eating as well.

Unfortunately, bears have free will, and regardless of what we eat, that bear could still attack.

Of Berries and Worms

When Sarah attended her first seminar with me, she scribbled "Luna," "photography," and "poison berries" in her notes. I have since revealed that I had a dog named Luna and enjoy photography, but I have yet to discuss the berries. This is a reference to an analogy I had been using to describe why negative memories are so much more salient than positive ones. It is really important to the brain, and the entire organism, to learn about all the great things in the world that may provide it with pleasure, but it is absolutely essential to learn what things may harm or kill it. The brain contains mechanisms to learn through both reward and punishment, and lessons learned by negative consequences are learned faster and more profoundly. Negative outcomes have a more significant impact on our immediate survival. Those are the poison berries.

The context of the berries goes as follows. Imagine the life of an early human being, exploring the world, collecting experiences, and learning about the wonders and dangers it has to offer. He may stumble onto a bush producing some delicious-looking berries and sample one or two. The berries taste great, and there appear to be no negative consequences, so he eats some more. They are refreshing, nutritious, and as it turns out, the sugar inside them helps energize the early human a bit, resulting in an increase in dopamine activity in the nucleus accumbens. It is important to remember that the berries of this bush are edible, and with a few repetitions his brain will most certainly remember that. The brain will also remember any stimuli that may be associated with the berries, such as the type of bush, location, time of day, climate, billboard advertisements, or any other markers that would inform a hungry brain on the trail that a potential meal is ahead. Remembering the tasty berries is adaptive.

On the other hand, imagine the early human stumbles onto a different bush covered in berries. This time upon sampling one or two, it makes him sick. Maybe it makes his companions sick as well, and some of them die. Although it is important to remember the good-tasting, nutritious berries, it is absolutely essential to remember the ones that may kill you. (Or which berries would make a good bear poison. You get the idea.)

Memories formed from negative experiences are far more influential on our behavior than memories formed solely from reward. For another example, consider how quickly we learn to not touch a hot pan on the stove when we accidentally burn ourselves as compared to simply being warned not to touch it. Lessons learned through first-degree burns are much more immediate than lessons learned through discussion.

Theoretically, the poison berries model can be used to reduce our cravings for the foods we would like to consume less often. If we can learn to associate negative consequences with their consumption, our brains produce less dopamine in the presence of the triggers and the urge is diminished. This is the basis of what is called aversion therapy. This can and does work, but its use with food is limited. There is a drug, Antabuse, that creates hangover symptoms immediately following the consumption of alcohol that uses this principle to help people stop drinking. However, everyone needs to continue eating. The method to losing weight is to eat less and eat healthier.

I went on a lot about doughnuts a few pages ago.[71] If, hypothetically, I could use some substance to make me nauseous every time I ate a doughnut, eventually my brain would reverse its opinion on doughnuts. The very sight of an ad for doughnuts would bring up negative associations, and I would be so repulsed by the idea of consuming them that I would gladly drive right by any and all doughnut shops as I enjoy a healthier life. That of course assumes that I use the substance reliably every time I eat a doughnut and remember to do so. Not only does such a substance not exist, I could not trust my brain to always administer it as needed. And would it even make sense to only target doughnuts, or would I have to target all pastries? What about candy bars and other snacks? Sugary drinks and ice cream? I am not sure I could handle that much artificially induced nausea. Even if a magic pill existed to help us, it is so damn difficult to change our behavior.

I do know of a few cases where people have accidentally "poison-

71 It just occurred to me that you find very few books about losing weight that talk in length about doughnuts.

berried" themselves into restricting their diets and therefore losing weight.

I know a little girl who once learned a joke typical of young kids, one of the variations on "What's grosser than gross?" jokes. It went like this: What's grosser than biting into an apple and finding a worm in it? Biting into an apple and finding half a worm in it.

When that little girl fully processed the meaning of that punchline, it severely turned her off from eating apples. It also turned her off from eating anything remotely resembling a worm, such as spaghetti or other noodles. It even completely turned her off from eating freshly plucked earthworms.

Eventually, she overcame her aversion to apples and pasta. She has yet to eat a worm.

Another case is a friend who explained to me how she gave up eating meat. She said she was driving to dinner when she passed the remains of a recent road kill. The image of the dead animal disturbed her, and she carried it in her head as she went into the restaurant. She suddenly made an association with the meat she was about to eat and the animal carcass she passed, and like that, meat was no longer appealing to her. From that day forward, she was a strict vegetarian.

By the way, a vegetarian diet is not necessarily conducive to weight loss. Chef Suzi Gerber covered this earlier, and it's also explained well by my friend comedian Cara Tramontano, who says, "Because there is no meat in a Snickers bar. Or five of them." But the diet does cut out a category of potential calories and promotes weight loss if the remaining calories taken in are healthy ones consumed in moderation.

I have another friend who gave up gluten because she started to experience stomach cramps and bloating after eating, and someone suggested she might be having a reaction to gluten. After cutting it out, she felt great. Then when she experimented with glutenous food, the cramps came back. So she is now convinced that the discomfort was due to gluten intolerance and refuses to consume any foods that are not gluten-free. Although weight loss was not the objective, this change has drastically reduced her consumption of breads, pastas, cereals, and yes, even doughnuts, leading indirectly to weight loss.

Like a vegetarian diet, a gluten-free diet is not necessarily low calorie. There is no gluten in potato chips, peanut butter, or bacon.

I had a similar experience that was caused by alcohol. At some point I started noticing discomfort after drinking beer, so naturally I cut back on it. However, my brain still seems to think it loves the taste of it, so every now and then I order one and am promptly reminded of how bad it makes me feel. It has gotten to the point that as I sit here writing this, I cannot remember the last time I had an alcoholic drink. I haven't quit drinking from a cognitive perspective, but I've effectively quit drinking from a behavioral one, and in the process I have been sparing myself all the extra calories in alcohol.

Cutting out alcohol significantly reduces my calorie intake, because it isn't just the calories in the alcohol, it's the calories I would consume because of the alcohol. Alcohol lowers inhibitions. It lowers the ability of the prefrontal cortex to suppress urges. For me, I learned that a beer or two at a comedy show increased the likelihood I would be pulling into a drive-through on the way home. Thankfully, beer now causes me abdominal pain. That's a strange sentence to think, let alone type, but I'm thankful for pain. Um, yay me.

Clearly, we can't afford to be grossed out or experience pain from everything we consume, but a scoop of metaphorical poison berries can help us change our habits.

Stress Eating Over a Caterpillar

One of the things we love about Montreal is that it is only about a forty-five-minute drive to the US border. This means we get to enjoy life in another country, removed from the day-to-day reminders of America, but when we need something from home we can always hop across the border. The closest American city is Plattsburgh, New York, which isn't the most interesting city to visit, but we are damn thankful for its existence. Occasionally we venture south to buy things we can't seem to find in Canada or send mail using the US postal system because international postage, even if crossing an imaginary line in the sand less than an hour away, is prohibitively expensive. We also visit the States for health care. We have nothing against the Canadian system, but because we spend most of our time touring the US, we maintain our American health insurance even during extended stays in Canada. We've been lucky not to need emergency services, at least until a few weeks ago.

Our daughter, Alyssa, has a scooter that she uses to get around the city faster and with more fun than walking. It was a nice sunny day in late June. A perfect day, really. The kind of day that makes it really hard for me to stay indoors and write.[72] To give me some space, Sarah decided to take Alyssa to a playground at the base of Mount Royal Park.[73] I barely had time to finish a few pages before my phone rang an hour later. It was Sarah, and they needed me to pick them up as soon as possible. Alyssa had an accident.

Immediately I closed up what I was doing, ran outside, and hopped into the car. Using Sarah's GPS coordinates, I found her on a sidewalk near a downed scooter and tending to our daughter. Alyssa had been scooting fast down a hill when she hit something in the sidewalk and fell. There was blood on both of them and a big cut above Alyssa's eyebrow. I helped them into the car and we left the scene.

Honestly, the injury did not look that serious at first, but when Sarah cleaned it up, we could see pretty deep into forehead flesh. Alyssa was no longer in pain, but Sarah and I knew we needed to get her extra face hole sewn up as soon as we could, so we hit the road for Plattsburgh. Not that I would encourage

---

72 Thankfully, today it is raining.

73 Montreal has a small mountain in the middle of it called Mount Royal, or *Mont Royal* in French, and saying that really fast is how the city got its name.

anyone to do this on purpose, but we found that having an injured five-year-old in need of medical care in the car really speeds up crossing the border.

We got to the emergency room and were instructed to wait. I predicted we would be there for a while and offered to make a Starbucks run for Sarah and me. With everything under control at the hospital, Sarah agreed, so I drove to the Plattsburgh Starbucks, one we'd visited plenty of times before, and ordered my usual cold brew because at that point in my night, I had already maxed out my calories for the day and a cold brew clocks in at under five. I know coffee normally has zero calories, that it is all the other stuff we add to make it palatable that beefs it up, but I never developed a taste for regular black coffee. Whatever the process is for making cold brew makes it smoother, and I can easily drink it without adding cream or sugar. Hell, I liked it before I started counting calories.

As I was sitting in the drive-through waiting on my order and thinking about what a calorie smart decision I'd made, I noticed that right across the street from me was a Taco Bell. A lot of people joke about the Bell, but I freaking love it. It is by far my favorite fast-food chain, and it remains so despite my having worked there for a year in college. Their food may not be authentic Mexican like your *abuela* makes, but it is damn tasty. Taco Bell had been on my mind recently in Montreal, as I'd had a craving one day and was surprised to learn that there are no longer any locations in the entire province of Quebec.[74] The closest one is in a city called

74 They were literally closed months before we got there! According to Selena Ross, "Au Revoir, Taco Bell: Chain Is Closing All Quebec Locations" (CTV News Montreal, January 7, 2022), https://montreal.ctvnews.ca/u-revoir-taco-bell-chain-is-closing-all-quebec-locations-1.5731928.

Hawkesbury, Ontario, about an hour and a half away. I may love the Bell, but I am not going to make a special trip to another province for a bean burrito with extra red sauce. Having one right next to me on this unexpected trip to America, well, that was an entirely different situation.

So, I'd been craving Taco Bell and I knew there wasn't one back home and my opportunities for having it again were limited, but I also knew I had already eaten my daily allotment of calories. Still, as I sat in that Starbucks drive-through line, I couldn't shake the craving. As I collected my coffee order, I realized there was one more thing influencing my thought process that I hadn't considered: stress. I was holding together fine, but my daughter's accident, her injury, and this impromptu trip to the emergency room had me extremely stressed. I knew my cravings were partially stress-based, even as I drove my ass to the Taco Bell and ordered two tacos and a bean burrito, extra red sauce.

My daughter needed my calm mind more than a slightly skinnier daddy that night.

When I returned to the hospital I found that Alyssa had been taken to a treatment room and was being administered analgesics, otherwise known as painkillers. Sarah and I stood by as they prepped her for stitches, and she handled it like the brave little girl we know her to be. When it was all over, she had five stitches above her eyebrow, which she thought resembled a caterpillar. She thought it looked cool. And you know what? Her caterpillar looked totally cool.

Shark Mode

If I could lose weight under ideal circumstances, I would go away to a remote cabin for six months by myself with nothing but a fifty-pound bag of dried beans and some hot sauce to sustain me. Just drive me out to the middle of nowhere, miles from the nearest restaurant, outside the range of any delivery service, and leave me there. Not because I need the solitude, or because of all the exercise I would hypothetically get chopping my own firewood every day, but because when I am deprived of sufficient calories, I can be a real asshole to the people around me.

I'm usually an extremely nice guy, but trust me, I can be insufferable.

I don't envy anyone who has to spend time with me when I am calorie-deprived. Unfortunately, by virtue of not yet being self-sufficient, my daughter has no choice but to be in my life. On the other hand, Sarah has volunteered to share her life with me. She is free to leave if she wants, and the fact that she chooses not to sometimes amazes me.

"Hangry" is a word that has been growing in popularity, and it perfectly describes an unfortunate side effect of restricted consumption. I guess because "being a miserable dick" wouldn't look good on a Snickers label.

Hunger doesn't necessarily make me angry, but being hungry exaggerates my responses to things that may otherwise only slightly annoy or irritate me. I am an easygoing guy. Hell, I literally wrote the book on taking it easy, and usually I have no problem shrugging off minor annoyances. But man, when the blood sugar is low, I can get agitated over the slightest little thing, and no matter how much you may love your family, there are always little things. I absolutely adore my daughter, and I am completely in love with Sarah, but this week in particular, both of them have been pissing me off. I find myself snapping at them with very little provocation and getting all worked up over the stupidest shit. Not coincidentally, this week I have also been really good about keeping my calorie count down.

There is no need for the details, but this morning I woke up realizing how insufferable I must have been and immediately apologized to them both. Sarah told me that she and Alyssa had discussed it in private, explaining that Daddy had been getting cranky because of his diet. My daughter said that when I was irritable, I was in "shark mode," and she knows when to stay away from the shark. Although I think that is hella cute, I wish none of us had to endure this. I wish I could be my usual, happy self all the time, but this is another hurdle I need to get over if I am going to get fit.

At least I have lost a few more pounds this week, so there is a silver lining to being such a prick.

Not everyone who restricts their calories gets hangry, and not everyone who gets hangry is hangry the whole time they're restricting, but hanger is a real phenomenon. As I have previously discussed, the prefrontal cortex is the home of conscious thought, and it has the ability to control impulses from other areas of the brain. If those impulses are coming from the amygdala, then we are talking about emotional regulation. As most owners of fully functioning brains know, we are able to modify, suppress, or redirect our emotional responses to fit the needs of the situation we find ourselves in. Schoolkids try not to laugh when the teacher tells them to be quiet.[75] We hold back our tears to appear strong to those who depend on us or to mask our vulnerabilities. We suppress anger in certain social settings to avoid causing a scene. We regulate our emotions as frequently as we experience them, and to do that the prefrontal cortex needs fuel in the form of calories. Specifically, the calories that come from sugar.

Without sufficient fuel, the prefrontal cortex cannot function properly. Not just with regulating emotions, but we have difficulties thinking clearly, we make bonehead decisions, and we become more prone to acting out of habit. We also get light-headed, klutzy, or impatient. The brain is a big old machine consisting of two pounds of fat and some other stuff, and it needs sugar to work properly. The brain actually uses half of the body's sugar energy.

Obviously, we all need our prefrontal cortex working well. Nearly everything I do professionally demands that my brain, specifically my prefrontal cortex, has a full tank of the sweet stuff. For example, in my first year as a public speaker, I learned that I should never give seminars on an empty stomach. I had a few mornings in the beginning when I skipped breakfast in favor of sleeping an extra twenty minutes. Not only was I less energetic, but it became harder to communicate effectively and keep my ideas straight. Now whenever I am on the circuit, I make sure every hotel stay

75 An example I know far too well.

comes with a decent breakfast option. These are the lessons you learn on the road. Never skip breakfast. As a bonus tip, invest in wrinkle-free shirts. I also never perform comedy while hungry, another lesson I learned the hard way. Comedians can bomb—it is something that all of us experience and get used to. I don't bomb often, but when it happens, I would rather bomb because my jokes suck than bomb because I forgot them or couldn't think clearly. Whether I'm in a conference room or at a comedy club, standing in front of a room full of people is the last place I want to experience brain fog.

Sarah and I have already shared bits and pieces of the story of how we started dating. I mentioned that we met for dinner in Tampa, where she was working temporarily, two days before a comedy show in her hometown of Gainesville. Well, after we went our separate ways, I spent a day exploring Tampa, shooting photos around town and across the bay in St. Petersburg. I toured the Salvador Dalí Museum, took in all the wonderful murals of the arts district, and somehow forgot to eat before heading north to Gainesville. I think I may have been running late. When I made it to the club, I parked my car and quickly went to check in with the manager. Once I settled in, I noticed that my head wasn't right. I was feeling loopy, which I recognized as a symptom of low blood sugar. I needed to eat something before I got onstage and bombed. There was a pizza joint across the street, and as I rushed over to grab a slice of brain fuel, I saw Sarah walking toward me on her way to surprise me at the show. To this day, this is one of my favorite memories of Sarah, walking toward me after she had driven up from Tampa to watch me perform. Sarah joined me at the pizza place. I ate a slice, maybe two, and quickly regained the full functioning of my brain. We walked back across the street, and when it was my time to perform, I freaking killed it.

After the show, Sarah went home and I walked back to my car with my friend Lisa, who was putting me up that night. I reached for my keys as we approached and was horrified when I realized I did not have them. We soon found them, in the ignition of my car. In my hypoglycemic state, I must have locked myself out, locked my keys in, and left the lights on to drain the battery for good measure. Thankfully, Lisa was willing to wait for a tow truck with me. The brain needs sugar, yo.

Still, I'd rather lock myself out of my car, drain the battery, and have to sit and wait for help than get disproportionately angry at my family.

As an aside, I've discussed how the brain is made of fat, uses dissolved salt to generate electricity, and uses sugar to fuel the whole process. Fat, salt, and sugar. Three things that we are often told are bad for us are actually essential to the health and functioning of the brain. Naturally, the brain is all about self-preservation, and one way to ensure there will always be a supply of fat, salt, and sugar is to make them all taste good as ingredients in food. Individually they may not be so appealing, as I don't think I would enjoy a spoonful of lard or a heaping pile of salt by itself, but together they are a winning combination. Man, now I'm craving potato chips. Food that tastes good also stimulates dopamine activity in the nucleus accumbens, helping our brain to remember, and eventually repeat, the behaviors that provide us with lots of fat, salt, and sugar. If I had a bag of chips available at the moment, I would most likely be absent-mindedly snacking on them and probably wouldn't stop until I hit the bottom of the bag. The problem, of course, is that throughout human evolution, until relatively recently, we never encountered fat, salt, and sugar in such abundance to the point that consuming too much of one became unhealthy. But today we do, and they are bad for us in large enough doses.

Another thing happens when we are calorie-deprived: we get stressed. We may not identify the way we feel as stress, but that is what happens to us internally. I previously explained how stress is our brain's reaction to a perception of threat. Well, an absence of fuel is considered a threat by the brain. It's not a bear but something way worse. The brain needs fuel to do more than think clearly. It needs fuel to help sustain its very existence, so of course it responds to deprivation as if it is under attack. When the brain is starving, it reacts like it would to any other threat triggering the autonomic nervous system and causes some familiar physiological changes, engaging our fight-or-flight[76] response and cranking out cortisol. I bet some of the potentially aggressive behaviors we are likely to express while in that state will help us get fed.

And if we are in that already heightened state and something ticks us off . . . we enter shark mode.

My daughter is a really good kid, but from now on, whenever Alyssa misbehaves or needs to be redirected, I'll warn her that I'm going to *unleash the shark*!

76 I always imagine someone annoyingly shouting, "Don't forget 'freeze'!" when I read this line.

Eating or Screwing?

If you are my mom, you may want to skip this part.

I studied sexual behavior in graduate school; it was my primary research interest. Part of the reason I chose that path was that I was really interested in sex, the behavior. As in having it. At some point in college, as a young academic mind, I realized I had the freedom to study whatever subject caught my interest. What could be more interesting than sex? For me, nothing.

Most people enjoy sex, and most people are interested in sex, but few people devote their research to sex. At least, that was how I might have explained it if we had met at a bar in my twenties. Now, I can't say that my current sex drive is higher than most, but I do think when I was younger it was higher than average. A lot of people might think that about themselves, but I had data to back my claim. In my research, I used surveys to measure sexual desire and motivation, and when I scored myself[77] on these same instruments, I often placed higher than average.

Let me put it this way: most people enjoy eating, and most people are interested in good food, but few people make it to the four hundred club. As I've touched on previously, sex and eating are intricately linked, as both stem from closely related structures in the brain and both contribute to the survival of our species. Of

---

77 Clearly having knowledge of the survey instrument would influence my results, but I tried to be as honest as I could to myself, and my scores weren't used for research.

the two behaviors, eating is more important to individual survival and is a socially acceptable public activity, so naturally we do more eating than screwing.

Also, screwing uses a lot of energy, especially when you do it right, which is one reason stress, and the cortisol it produces, also knocks out our sex drive. You don't want to suddenly get the urge to engage in sexual behavior when you are being attacked by a bear. Using a lot of energy leads to a need to replenish, so screwing in turn leads to eventual eating. However, eating doesn't necessarily lead to screwing. It is reasonable to say that the more we eat, the less we screw. This was certainly the case for me. Over the years, there have been many nights when after a big meal, even on a date, all I wanted to do was crawl into my bed and use it for sleeping. As foods that are high in carbohydrates have mood-elevating qualities, if we are experiencing a dry spell and feeling a little lonely as a result, we might be drawn to improve our mood with snacks. In other words, the less we screw, the more we eat. The more we eat, the less we screw.

As relationships progress, it is common for couples to gain weight together. This has definitely been my experience with Sarah and in almost every serious relationship I have ever had. If you listen to enough stand-up comedy, you'll eventually get the impression that comedians think nothing kills a sex drive like marriage. I think for a lot of couples, the more time they spend together the more eating and less screwing they are doing. There is a point where the phrase "Netflix and chill" literally becomes watching Netflix and then falling asleep. All of this is why I never thought to question it as my sex drive was diminishing. Sure, Sarah and I still managed to have an active sex life—we even made a baby as proof—but my weight gain made me much less active than I had been in the past, and much less physical and flexible.

It was easy to blame the decline on getting older. I was also aging, and the stand-up comics all seem to agree that getting older kills boners. Luckily, I managed to enter middle age in the time of Viagra, something for which I could not be more thankful, but Viagra doesn't give you the energy you need to keep you going. Viagra doesn't prevent your back from hurting or your legs from cramping. Viagra certainly doesn't make you less heavy when on top of your partner. Viagra also doesn't increase desire; it just makes erections stronger and helps you keep them longer.

However, as I started losing weight, my drive started coming back, first in the form of increased fantasies, then greater desire, more energy, and more stamina. I am now in my early fifties, and although I am nowhere near where I was in my twenties or thirties, I feel like I could hold my own in a room full of forty-year-old men. Provided there are some women in that room. Losing nearly one hundred pounds has brought a great deal of my sex drive back. I wonder what losing the rest of the weight is going to do.

I never thought I had to make a choice between eating or screwing, but logically speaking, if you do too much of the first, it gets in the way of the second. Sometimes it's literally in the way: have you ever tried to hold your belly back for some doggy style?[78] It ain't easy.

I am now at a body weight that is lower than where I was when Sarah and I first met, and I am damn happy to be experiencing

---

78 Sorry, Mom. I did tell you to skip this part.

the changes in my sex drive and performance that go along with that. Sex is healthy, and losing weight has made me healthier in so many ways.

4

The Eye-Opening Event

Throughout my years as a public speaker, I have given a lot of talks about behavior change. Much as I have done here, I explain some of the reasons why change is so difficult and why so few of us are successful in changing our behavior for the long term. Old habits, learned through a process of reinforcement, are hard to break. This is why my brain continues to love doughnuts and often experiences the urge to get them. New habits seem less rewarding in comparison. My brain is still learning to enjoy healthier options, but I doubt I will crave kale anytime soon. Perhaps our old habits were learned because they were easier to obtain, and new ones may require greater effort. My brain loves when I am sitting on the couch, which is comfortable and relaxing, especially when compared to getting my ass outside for a jog. Change involves automating new behaviors and, unfortunately, most of our brains have already learned how to produce all the highly rewarding, low effort-behaviors by adulthood. Anything new is going to require some serious effort.

Often I am asked how to motivate someone to change, and my answer is always that you really can't. People absolutely have the capacity to change, there is no question about that, and I've provided myself, Sarah, and several other people as examples throughout this book, but they have to want to change on their own. There is very little we can do to inspire behavioral change in others without their own motivation.

Part of the problem is the relatively small incremental gain associated with behavior change. Sure, I could drive by the doughnut shop without succumbing to my inner struggle, but in the morning, I'll still wake up fat. What's the point of depriving myself if it doesn't immediately change my pants size? I see this same logic in smokers who know that in the long term smoking is bad for them, but this next cigarette is probably not going to give them cancer. To successfully change our behavior and achieve whatever goal we have set for ourselves, we need to repeatedly choose the healthy option despite the lack of immediate returns, and that requires internal conscious motivation.

Or external rewards that are great enough to be compelling. I love this quote[79] from *It's Always Sunny in Philadelphia* actor Rob McElhenney on how he once lost over sixty pounds: "All you need to do is lift weights six days a week, stop drinking alcohol, don't eat anything after 7 p.m., don't eat any carbs or sugar at all, in fact just don't eat anything you like, get the personal trainer from *Magic*

---

79 As posted to his Instagram on September 5, 2018, https://www.instagram.com/p/BnXtEz1BLFP.

Mike, sleep nine hours a night, run three miles a day, and have a studio pay for the whole thing over a six to seven-month span. I don't know why everyone's not doing this. It's a super realistic lifestyle and an appropriate body image to compare oneself to."

It is unfortunate, but sometimes it takes extreme circumstances to motivate change. Often people do not seriously commit to a healthier lifestyle until their life is threatened. Bears can be very motivating. I know smokers who were able to quit after a cancer scare or after surviving cancer. Alcoholics and other addicts are sometimes motivated to change their behavior after hitting rock bottom. Surviving a heart attack or stroke can be a real eye-opening event.

I have never suffered such an extreme event, but when Sarah convinced me to get a physical before becoming a dad, my eyes were not only opened wide but squeegeed clean. I always knew that I had to lose weight, but I couldn't believe I had let myself hit four hundred pounds. My blood pressure was dangerously high, heart attack or stroke high. I realized that, holy shit, I was quite literally near death if I didn't start making some immediate changes.

Thankfully I avoided an extreme illness, but this was my eye-opening event. As we discussed my condition, all of the symptoms that had been creeping up on me over the years came to light. My legs and ankles were abnormally swollen, my joints suffered from inflammation. My sex drive had significantly reduced, which perhaps wasn't that bad given my overall energy levels had greatly diminished, but damn it, I love sex! I had a beautiful, sexy red-headed wife with a perfect waist-to-hip ratio, and my body wasn't functioning like it should. Sex, although incredibly important, was just one part of my life; the reality was that I felt terrible all the time.

Sarah and I used to have a running joke between us: "free condo." It was based on the fact that when we purchased our home in Montreal, we were told that if one of us dies before the mortgage is fully paid, the bank will pay off the remaining balance. Therefore, the survivor would get a free condo. Shortly after we signed the paperwork, anytime one of us (usually me) would do something stupid like not wear a seat belt or announce that we were going to eat a seventy-two-ounce steak in Amarillo (but . . . if I eat it in an hour, it's free!), the other would simply turn and say, "I guess I'm getting that free condo," and we'd rethink our stupid life choice.

This physical exam successfully took the humor out of that joke by making the free condo seem like a very real possibility for Sarah. Thankfully, I didn't just leave that clinic with a stack of bad news. I left with motivation, and some insight into sleep apnea, which would ultimately help kick-start my weight loss. My daughter was born a month later, and I have been struggling to get healthy ever since.

The "Not-So-Secret" Secret

OK, so how exactly am I doing it? Every time I post a new photo to social media, at least one person comments or sends me a private message asking what I am doing to lose the weight.

If you have read this far, then it should be no secret that there is no secret. I have been doing precisely what I have always claimed we all already know to do. I have been eating less and exercising more. That's it. Calories in, calories out. No special program, no secret technique, just good old-fashioned, traditional wisdom coupled with a greater sense of motivation from a now five-year-old daughter with whom I want to spend as much time as I possibly can.

It really is that simple. You may recall that earlier I mentioned that it may be simple, but it ain't easy. It has definitely not been an easy road to get to where I am. There have been lots of bumps along the way, whether they were the circumstances of being on tour, the stress associated with the pandemic, holidays and other celebrations involving food, or just plain relapses. My weight has fluctuated a lot over the past five years, but at least when I plot it on a graph, I see a general downward slope and that feels great. I understand that whenever people ask me how I am losing weight, what they are really wondering is how I am managing to eat less and exercise more.

Let me start with eating less.

Despite personal preferences, I think everyone can agree that human beings are omnivorous. We can, and do, eat a variety of foods sourced from both plants and animals. Many people might choose to exclude one category or another,[80] but as a species we are built to eat it all. And we do. Unless it is poisonous, if there is a plant or animal in the world, somebody somewhere has figured out a way to eat it. We even figure out ways to eat some of the poisonous ones too. For example, Sarah is fond of making rhubarb crisp thanks to the availability of fresh rhubarb at the Montreal farmers markets.[81] Most of the rhubarb plant is toxic to humans, but luckily, some of our hungry ancestors figured out which part was safe to eat.

It should be understood that it isn't just that human beings are capable of eating a variety of foods but that we seek variety as part of our nature. Our bodies require a lot of different nutrients and not every food source contains them all, so we are naturally driven to consume different things. When we restrict our diet by going on a diet, we are behaving in a way that is against our natural tendency. As so many of us know through personal experience, that way of life is rarely sustainable. Diets, generally speaking, don't work.

Another thing I was first exposed to in Dr. Singh's class was that because of our need for diversity in foods, if we severely restrict our consumption to limit our variety, we will eventually lose weight. Even though most diets are not overly restrictive, when

---

80 Usually animal products. I have yet to meet a single person who refuses to eat plant matter.

81 Rhubarb crisp is amazing and Sarah showed me that it is really easy to make. Spoiler alert: the recipe is definitely not low-calorie

we decide to eat a smaller selection of foods, all diets will appear to work in the short-term. However, without introducing variety, our brain becomes less and less interested in consuming those limited options. We become bored with our food and eat less as a result. For most of us, a diet that restricts us to a single food type will not last long. Imagine a diet that consists of eating nothing but candy. Eventually, perhaps after some immediate weight gain, our brain would become less and less interested in candy and as a result we would start to lose weight. Candy is awesome, but candy does not contain all of the nutrients our body needs, and so its appeal would be diminished. I have seen this play out with my daughter (and her dad) after each Halloween. On the first night, the candy is novel and faces are stuffed, but the next day the candy seems less interesting and fewer pieces are consumed. Each day that goes by sees less and less candy action until eventually the bucket of treats gets neglected for so long it starts writing a manifesto.[82] Does this mean I recommend an all-candy diet to lose weight? Hell no, but I think you get how virtually any restriction on our variety will contribute to weight loss, at least until we go off the diet.

Ever stare into a stocked refrigerator and think that you have nothing to eat? I suspect that sensation reflects our need for variety, as the regularly consumed foods have lost their appeal.

I can remember Dr. Singh discussing wheat. Wheat is a grass used to produce flour, which has become a staple of foods throughout the world. Obviously, wheat flour is a good source of carbohydrates, but one of its real advantages is that it is resistant to spoiling. A sack of wheat can remain edible over an entire

---

82 As I write this, we still have way too much leftover candy from last Halloween.

winter, which was particularly important to humans living in parts of the world with seasonal changes before we developed a global economy. Imagine a family living in Europe back in the day and managing their food supply during the winter. There were no fresh fruits and vegetables available for consumption, but every night they could cook up a scoop of wheat.[83] After several days of eating wheat, imagine how bored they would be. I think on day five I'd be ready to pass.

So those wheat-eating humans figured out ways to trick their brains into thinking they were eating a variety of foods by changing its texture. Oh, you are bored with porridge and gruel? Perhaps you would be interested in a recipe we picked up from Italy called spaghetti. Tired of spaghetti? How about some tortellini or fettucine? Oh, I know, maybe you'd be interested in this new food called bread. We have a wide variety of types to choose from. How about a pancake, or maybe some pizza? The reason so many of our foods are wheat or other staple grains repackaged is our brain needs to think it is consuming variety. By the way, after you eat your wheat, there is some delicious wheat for dessert.

At least flour has a good number of calories in it to fuel a typical human's energy needs. However, the fewer the calories, the quicker our need for variety will kick in. Ever sit down and stuff your face with an entire head of iceberg lettuce? No dressing, nothing else, just lettuce. Maybe a single head isn't enough to completely satisfy our appetite. How about two? Three? Keep 'em coming, I have a Costco card. It is hard to imagine being completely satisfied with

---

83 When we traveled up to Dawson City in the Yukon, I found it interesting to learn that to avoid mass starvation during the Klondike Gold Rush of 1896 to 1899 each person making the trip had to bring enough food for an entire year. That included four hundred pounds of flour per person.

nothing but lettuce or celery because they lack certain nutrients our body needs to be able to function and survive, but it's also because humans have a relatively small stomach capacity. We only have so much space inside us devoted to digesting food, and if we fill it full of nutrient-poor lettuce, that lettuce is going to be taking up space when we encounter something more nutrient-dense. Many herbivores, like cows, have four stomachs to increase their capacity. We have one. Our brain needs to be smart about what it puts in there, and so our natural tendency is to seek a wide variety of calorie-rich foods.

By the way, buffets capitalize on this. I will admit that the lure of variety has gotten me in to more buffets than I care to remember. I love a good buffet,[84] and there are so many great ones in America, but I have had to drastically cut down on them in my quest to lose weight. This is one reason why I don't think I'll be going on any cruise ships for a while.

To be fair, I don't think any diet commonly suggested for weight loss is based on restricting someone to a single food, but I think it is helpful to understand we have an instinctive drive to consume variety. If we work within that framework, we can be a lot more successful in the long run.

When I tried vegetarianism, and even veganism, I had significant results. As a college student in Austin, the birthplace of Whole Foods, I found it easy to maintain a vegetarian lifestyle and saw a dramatic weight loss as a result. When I returned to eating animal products, I put the weight back on and then some over

---

84 How is this for irony: I remember a time when I was so big that I did not fit into a booth to eat at a buffet. I have no idea why that moment was not my "eye-opening event," but it wasn't. I moved to another table, with movable chairs, and proceeded to chow down.

the course of a couple of years. Because I have no moral objection to eating animals, I decided that this lifestyle would not be very sustainable for me.

I know plenty of people who have lost weight eating high-protein diets. I love meat, so this definitely has its appeal, as I could theoretically eat only steak. I am even very outspoken about my love of barbeque in my stand-up act. But the reality is that I don't think I can truly give up all my delicious carbs.

Plus, I like to have options. In the late nineties, it was easy to be a vegetarian living in Austin. There were specialty grocery stores, lots of vegetarian and vegan cafés, and almost all the restaurants in the central part of the city had plenty of vegetarian options. However, when I moved to New Orleans and was living near campus, I found it very difficult to keep up the lifestyle. I ended up eating a lot of peanut butter and jelly sandwiches, which were way more caloric than a plate of grilled shrimp or chicken.

I knew that whatever diet I was going to adopt, it had to include variety and allow for options. I settled on a relatively low-carbohydrate and low-fat diet, but rather than restricting myself to certain foods or depriving myself, I instead chose to count calories. I have been trying to keep my calories to under one thousand a day,[85] which is lower than the average body needs to sustain itself and certainly lower than a four-hundred-pound body needs,[86] and as a result I have been steadily losing weight.

---

85 This is a choice, not a recommendation. A lot of professionals recommend twelve hundred calories a day, but individual bodies have different needs. My allotment is only two hundred calories off from that recommendation, but I wouldn't suggest that you follow my lead without first checking with your doctor to learn what would work for you.

86 According to one calculator, with a sedentary lifestyle I required 3,268 calories a day just to sustain myself at my peak weight.

Yes, I slip up. Yes, I have accidental relapses and my weight bounces up and down, but overall, I have been sticking to or coming back to my one-thousand-calorie-a-day limit, and gradually I have been losing the weight. I use an app on my smartphone called Lose It![87] to log my calories whenever I eat. I find this system to be easy to manage, as I always have my phone on me and already spend a lot of time staring at it. As long as I'm going to have it in my hand anyway, I might as well use it to help me get healthy.

Like my friend Andrew Ginsburg suggested, I try to focus on lean proteins. I eat a lot of grilled chicken and fish. Turkey burgers are an amazing substitute for more caloric beef, and I find a can of tuna meat doused in calorie-free hot sauce makes a delicious and quick snack.

I should expand a little on the joys of hot sauce. Most are vinegar-based, which has practically no calories, and the flavor is enough to trick my brain into thinking it's something more substantial. I'll admit that there have been plenty of times when my cravings were satisfied simply by dousing a few drops of hot sauce directly on my tongue. I often stock a few different types of hot sauce, as different ones tend to pair better with different foods. In my opinion, Louisiana (the brand, not the state) hot sauce is best for tuna, and the Mexican sauce Chamoy is crazy delicious on popcorn as well as when used as a salad dressing.

Similarly, mustard and pickles are relatively calorie-free and help to stimulate the taste buds enough to fool the brain. Powdered flavorings like Montreal steak seasoning do the same trick. I'll sprinkle that or Tony Chachere's Creole Seasoning on just about anything but ice cream.

---

87 I am sure there are others that are just as helpful.

Fruits are great and surprisingly lower in calories than I sometimes expect them to be.[88] Vegetables are wonderful and filling, provided they are consumed as part of a salad. If I put enough variety in my salad, I can eat nothing but vegetables for a day. As often as I can, I'll make a big salad starting with a lettuce mix, adding tomatoes, sliced peppers, cucumbers, and whatever other vegetables we happen to have lying around. It'll feed me for a couple of days, and I will almost always see the impact on the scale.

Whenever available, I get light versions of everyday food products. Stuff like light mayonnaise, salad dressing, vegetarian baked beans (no pork), and skim milk. If there is something I want and a lower-fat or light option exists, I will always go for that instead.

The one exception to that rule is artificial sweetener. I don't enjoy it, and I think for many of the people who do, it is an acquired taste. I would rather do without sugar than consume artificial sweeteners. Sarah enjoys Stevia, but it just reminds me of the much better-tasting sugar I could be consuming.

Coffee and tea are calorie-free, and both seem to help quench my appetite. I love a good iced coffee, and a splash of skim milk has so few calories that I usually don't bother to add them to the count. Iced tea will always be my casual beverage of choice, and although I do have fond memories of southern-style sweet tea, I have successfully weaned myself off of it. By the way, for some reason Canada does not have real iced tea.[89] I know, I don't get it either. If you order iced tea at a restaurant in Canada, you'll get

---

88 It still amazes me every time I log some watermelon that it is only forty-five calories a cup.

89 We have discovered that neither does Australia or England. It's odd—they have plenty of tea and plenty of ice, but they have yet to figure out how to combine these two ingredients.

that artificial syrupy concoction that is typically sold at soda fountains.[90] Iced tea bags are not sold in grocery stores either, making it the one product I make sure we have plenty of whenever we cross the border north.

Ultimately with counting calories, it really doesn't matter what I eat as long as I stick to my calorie limit. Some days, I will indulge in a big breakfast, blowing my calories early on and then eating light to make up the difference later. This approach has helped me to lose weight without feeling deprived or restricted in any way.

Another thing calorie counting has done for me is teach me how to assess calories by sight. I can roughly estimate what I am going to consume at any meal, and usually I am fairly close. My stomach has been trained to be satisfied with 250- to 500-calorie meals, which is a far cry from the staggering calorie count per meal that I used to consume on a regular basis.

In addition, I can always find something I can eat wherever I may be. This was one of the harder things I experienced trying to be a vegetarian or vegan on the road.

Alcohol, on the other hand, is something that I have effectively given up. It wasn't intentional, and started with my drinking less and less frequently, but now I rarely have a drink anymore. There are a lot of calories in alcohol, and I am happy not consuming them. Plus, as a drug, alcohol loosens inhibitions. It makes it harder for my prefrontal cortex to monitor my behavior and prevent me from eating a bunch of other crap. I do love the taste of a good beer and a nice Bloody Mary, but I am OK without them.

---

90 We did find one restaurant in Niagara Falls, Ontario, that served real iced tea. It was amazing.

That is a basic rundown of what I've been doing, which is focused on counting calories. I have heard from lots of people who have had success with intermittent fasting, a diet that also allows for a variety of foods and flexibility, but I like counting calories because it is helping me learn how to eat better, smarter meals. Of course, it is hard to maintain any behavioral changes, which is why it has taken me so long and I have not yet reached my ultimate goal. Changing one's behavior is not easy, but there are things that I do, that anyone can do, to help the process.

A lot of diets fail because they focus on eliminating a form of reward—in this case food—from life. If weight loss is a goal, then some elimination is required, but if we don't replace that form of reward with something else, we are bound to relapse. I try to fill my life with rewarding activities as much as possible to provide my brain with alternative sources of dopamine. For example, instead of sitting around doing nothing and resisting the urge to eat out of boredom, I try to go for a walk or tour a museum that I have never been to. On days when that is not possible, I engage my hobbies, of which there are many, to keep my brain stimulated. I might work on my photography, which not only involves taking photos but also editing digitally, or I make other art; I think you are aware that I am also something of a writer. Sarah is a tango dancer, but she also enjoys making pottery at home. Any activity that your brain finds rewarding can be helpful in reducing the tendency to eat out of habit. When my hobbies are not enough, or I am no longer interested or able to engage them, I learn something new. During the pandemic, we had to find lots of new ways to occupy our lives for many reasons, not just weight loss, and that is when

I started to turn my attention to filmmaking. I am quite proud of some of my videos, and making more is something I can do with Sarah and Alyssa.[91]

What I have just described is often referred to by psychologists as reward substitution. Like when I described meeting Sarah, how my brain was content to substitute the reward of eating dinner for the more desirable reward of getting her naked.

Another thing that helps with any behavior change is modifying my thoughts, and in this case, it is modifying my thoughts about food. Reframing is a cognitive technique that simply refers to changing the way we think about our behavior and the outcomes. For example, I may think doughnuts are delicious, and the reality is that they are, but I can learn to think about them differently. They are, after all, fried balls of wheat. Or, more specifically, fried balls of bread covered with some sugar and maybe stuffed with some jelly. That may still be an appetizing combination, but it sounds less appealing and therefore easier to pass up than, oh man, doughnuts!

Or maybe I rethink how much of a rare treat it really is. The key to my doughnut story earlier was that when living in San Francisco, I perceived going to Krispy Kreme as a rare opportunity, but the reality was that I could go any day, at any time, because I owned and had full-time access to a car. Any time I wanted, I could hop in the car and take a trip to grab some doughnuts, and as I came to think about it as more of a mundane experience and less special, my desire to eat them while driving south on the 280 was diminished.

---

91 From a very early age I wanted to be involved with film. I remember making a pact with a friend in elementary school that someday we would meet again in Hollywood. When I finally did move there, I sometimes wondered if he followed through as well.

I have written about a lot of the foods that I love in this book, mostly to make points, but the truth is that in order to lose the weight I have had to adjust the way I think about them. Poutine, although delicious, really isn't all that special, and therefore I have successfully avoided it for most of the summer. I may not have direct access to my nucleus accumbens to alter the dopamine released with each bite of doughnut or plate of poutine, but I can reduce their appeal by changing the activity of the prefrontal cortex. The more I change my thoughts, the more my thoughts factor into my automatic behavioral choices. In other words, I can reduce my tendency to express certain habits by changing the way I think about them.

At the same time, I can reduce the impact that triggers have on my behavior. When our brain learns about a source of reward, like doughnuts, it also learns how to predict that reward by remembering anything associated with the reward. Driving down Interstate 280 and passing billboards for Krispy Kreme were triggers causing my brain to crave doughnuts. Sometimes these associations inspire urges that become difficult to resist. We can retrain those associations or learn new ones.

I travel a lot, and just as I associate poutine with Montreal, there are foods that I associate with almost every place I go. I associate New York City with bagels and pizza, Austin with bowls of chili con queso,[92] Vermont with ice cream, Philadelphia with cheesesteaks, Kansas City with barbeque ribs, Texas with barbeque brisket, the Carolinas with barbeque pork, Milwaukee and the entire Midwest with loaded Bloody Marys, Salt Lake City

92 Seriously, Austin has some of the best queso.

with dirty sodas (imagine mixing cocktails but with soft drinks and adding extra sugar), and Chicago with deep-dish pizza (which my friend and fellow New Yorker Rigel disparagingly refers to as "pasta cake"). Enjoying each of these treats once in a while is not a big deal, but when I found myself constantly traveling and repeatedly visiting these places, I found myself eating a bit much every time. By engaging in new and different experiences as I travel, I have been actively reducing the associations made by my brain. Like with doughnuts, I am slowly convincing my brain that just because I am in a certain place does not mean I have to partake in a certain high-calorie food.

Now let me address exercising more.

I will admit that I find it easier to eat less than to exercise more, and thankfully that seems to have helped me lose weight so far. My friends Andrew Ginsburg and Suzi Gerber both emphasized the importance of eating less to lose body weight, so I think I am doing OK. However, I do try to make sure I am burning a few more calories than I used to.

I find exercise difficult for a couple of reasons. First, it's boring. When I think of exercise, I think of going to a gym and either lifting weights or working out on some machine. Repetitious body movements are literally the definition of exercise, and my brain finds absolutely no joy in this. Andrew is a bodybuilder and actively enjoys lifting weights. I envy him for that, because for me, lifting weights only to put them back down and lift them again is one of the most boring activities I can imagine, and I can imagine quite a bit. Running on a treadmill? I'd rather sit and watch the Weather Channel.

Again, I can reframe the way I think about exercise. It doesn't have to be lifting weights or going to a gym. It can be going for a walk in a park or playing with my daughter. Exercise can be going on a bike ride or having sex. Any physical activity is exercise, and I can and do try to find activities that I enjoy. For the sake of my own motivation, I try not to think of them as exercise.

My favorite form of exercise, other than the obvious, is walking, and I try to go for a walk every day. Once again, my smartphone helps with this, as I have a pedometer installed on it. It tracks my steps and sends me nice reminders to prompt me to get off my ass if I have been too sedentary that day.

Another reason why exercise is difficult is that the excess body weight I have collected over the years of becoming a four hundred-pound man makes it sometimes painful to exercise. I lack the flexibility and stamina of my youth, but I have been finding that as I slim down, a lot of that is coming back. I suspect that the more weight I lose, the more exercise I will be able to incorporate into my life. And the more I will be able to keep my promise to Alyssa.

FAT TALES

Popcorn for Breakfast

I woke up over two hours ago. With the rest of my family still sleeping soundly, I spent the first hour of morning consciousness trying in vain to fall back asleep. Failing at that, I decided to get up and grab some breakfast, so I made my way to the kitchen. Waiting for me was a bowl of popcorn I had made last night to share with my daughter as we watched the movie *Paddington*. I remembered making it: I loaded it into the microwave, kept an eye on it as it popped, and took it out to cool before finding that, as I had hoped, the marmalade-eating bear with a British accent had put Alyssa to sleep. Feeling tired myself, I took that as my cue and put myself to bed, forgetting all about the fresh batch of popcorn that was now going to be my breakfast with a few dashes of hot sauce. Not a typical breakfast, but not super strange either. Marmalade? Now that's just gross.

It reminded me of a bit I hadn't used onstage in a long time.

> I was recently eating breakfast, and I noticed right there on the container of cookie dough, the words "Please do not consume raw cookie dough."
>
> Now, do you skinny people know another way to eat cookie dough that I'm not aware of? You take a bucket of dough, a spoon, and some depression . . . that's a meal!

It was an opener, meant to introduce my sarcastic and often self-deprecating sense of humor and acknowledge that I am a big guy. Sometimes, depending on audience reaction, I'd continue with a comment about the joke itself.

> I'm glad at least some of you recognized that as a joke, while the rest of you were like, "When you got onstage we were thinking, *This guy eats cookie dough for breakfast!*"

Like many of my jokes, it was inspired by some truth. Years ago, while living in San Francisco, I remember waking up one morning, stumbling into the kitchen, and scanning the fridge for a quick snack. There wasn't much, but I saw a container of chocolate chip cookie dough my former girlfriend had purchased, and without hesitating, I ripped it open and scarfed down a couple of heaping spoonfuls. As I finished, the idea of a fat guy eating cookie dough for breakfast amused me, and the bit was born. It was introduced at an open mic that night, and refined with repeated usage. Over time it became a good opener, helping me to quickly establish my onstage character. For the record, depression was not involved—we just hadn't gone shopping for a while.

After eating my breakfast popcorn, I decided to open my computer to use the time productively. It is now about 7:30 a.m.

It is a Sunday, specifically Father's Day, and I have no reason to be waking up so early. Later on, I am sure that Sarah and Alyssa have some celebratory plans in store for me, but nothing urgent made me get up at five in the morning. No gigs, no day job, no travel plans. I didn't fall asleep really early, I don't suffer from anxiety,[93] and there were no loud noises or anything. I didn't even have an alarm set. Nothing.

One of the first things I did when I started to work on my health was get treated for my sleep apnea. It had been previously undiagnosed, but when I went in for my eye-opening checkup, the doctor immediately identified me as someone suffering from sleep apnea. It took some time and some effort from Sarah, but later in the year I was able to do a sleep study and get fitted for a CPAP shortly after. Treating my sleep apnea was the first step in my road to recovery, and if I hadn't addressed it, none of my subsequent weight loss would have been possible.

I talked a lot about sleep apnea in *The Art of Taking It Easy*, so I don't want to cover it again here, but I strongly encourage anyone who suspects they may have an issue to get checked. After a little over four years of treatment, I have never slept better in my life.

And a good night's rest means an easier wake up. In fact, like today, I am often the first person awake in my home.

Old Habits Die Hard

I count calories. I find it incredibly useful to track what I have eaten throughout the day so that I can make sure I do not overeat.

93 It was the popcorn, man; it was calling me! How dare I waste food during a recession!

It takes effort, conscious effort, to remember to add up each meal or snack, entering it into my smartphone app or keeping a running total in my head. Calorie tracking has not yet become an automatic habit for me, not yet delegated to the nucleus accumbens, and when I need the processing power of my prefrontal cortex for other, more important tasks, I sometimes cut myself some slack. One of those tasks is driving long distances. When I'm behind the wheels of a car, I think it is more valuable to have my mind focused on the road than tabulating whatever I ate that day, so I give myself a pass.[94] As I do most of the driving when we travel, my family probably agrees with that decision.

It was a long drive from Texas to Montreal, and granted we didn't do it all in one day, but the last day of travel was brutal, and after we arrived all I wanted to do was sleep. I woke up at around 2 p.m. the next day. Groggy and stumbling, I made my way to the kitchen, where I saw that Sarah had already unpacked our car. We had no groceries, but instinctively I opened up the fridge to stare at its contents and saw that she had put in there a half-empty pack of meat sticks we'd picked up on the road. I grabbed the package and started nibbling on one, then another, then another.

And then it hit me—I am supposed to be counting calories today. I gave myself a pass while on the road, but I needed to get back into the practice. I turned the package over and saw the lettering "110 calories" per meat stick. In my morning haze, how many had I consumed? Three? Four? Five? I had no idea. I had eaten them without thinking about it. I had eaten them out of habit.

---

94 Of course, it is possible to eat healthy on the road, and for the most part I do, but sometimes the brain needs more fuel than celery sticks.

Just like those damn doughnuts I used to talk about.

This type of mindless eating is a big part of why many people, including myself, find it so damn difficult to lose weight or make any meaningful changes to our behavior. Often, our behavior isn't the product of conscious thought; it is the product of habit. Our bodies are biological machines, and it takes the conscious effort of a pilot to change the course; otherwise it is going to stick to the course as programmed. We may have a strong desire to change our behavior, we may know how to change our behavior, but unless we are actively thinking about it when it matters, we will have a very difficult time changing our behavior.

I estimated five meat sticks at 550 calories, way more than I wanted to start my day with, and promptly ran to the other room to write this down. The struggle is real.

FAT TALES

Time to Wear the Big Boy Pants

I still have a long way to go, but losing one hundred pounds, or nearly one hundred depending on the week, is no small accomplishment. As my body shrank, I had a chance to "go shopping in my own closet," as Sarah says. People don't gain weight overnight. It's not like we wake up one day, look in the mirror, and go, "Oh great, guess this means I'm going to have to develop a personality." It is a gradual process, and along the way many people, myself included, accumulate an assortment of clothes in various sizes as they keep adding more and more Xs in front of that L on the tag. I outgrew plenty of sizes in my rise to four hundred, but I held on to my smaller clothes in case I learned how to eat a salad once in a while. On the way down from when my shirts started to look more like they were made to cover my car instead of a person, I figured it was about time to hit the storage unit and downsize my wardrobe. I have never been so happy to wear old clothes.

I went to high school in the late eighties, which you can imagine led to some questionable personal fashion choices. I won't go into the details, but I was very much inspired by my musical influences. Imagine emulating the look of bands like The Cure, Love and Rockets, or Depeche Mode while running around in the Texas heat. Thankfully I outgrew that look, but one trend from that era that continues to linger on in my style preferences is baggy pants. Regardless of my body type I don't think I can ever go back to wearing tight or fitted jeans. It's a comfort thing; loose is definitely the way to go.

I like my jeans like I like my women: big and loose.[95] I am bringing this clothing preference up for a few reasons. The first is that I have realized over the years that loose-fitting clothes are part of the problem. They are growth enablers. When my clothes fit loosely, it is much harder to track when I've gained weight. The second reason is that I would like to issue a warning to anyone standing behind me if my belt fails. However, the main reason I

95 Please don't tell Sarah I wrote this.

am bringing this up is to give the following story some context.

I have never shared this story with anyone. Not that it is terribly embarrassing or private, but it isn't about the proudest moment of my life either. I think all overweight people have moments where their weight gain gets thrown in their face, and this is one of mine.

As I have mentioned, after I finished college in Austin, I moved around the country a few times for my career. I never intended to move back to Texas, but I would always visit when I could, which never seemed to be often enough. Thankfully, during my first year as a public speaker, my tour had me bouncing all over Texas. My brother still lived in the state, now in Dallas, and I had an opportunity to spend a long weekend with him. With both of their children in one spot, our parents decided to fly in and join the party for a nice little King family reunion. Fittingly, we decided to go up the Reunion Tower.

If you've never been to Dallas, you should know that it has one of the most beautiful and iconic skylines in the country, and one of the key ingredients is a giant Tootsie Pop–shaped structure known as the Reunion Tower. During the day it stands prominently at the edge of downtown, and at night it lights up with a programmable display with all sorts of designs. At the top, there was a revolving restaurant that offered a panoramic view of the city from 560 feet in the sky for the cost of a cocktail. Even with all the years I spent in Texas, I had never been up there, and neither had anyone else in my family, so I suggested we go. It was summer in Texas, and I had on a baggy pair of cargo shorts, which I quickly found out were against the dress code of the swanky revolving cocktail bar overlooking Dallas. *No big deal,*

I thought. I was on tour, so I had my suitcase in the car. I sent my family up the elevator and went to change into some more respectable attire.

I went to the car, a large SUV I'd rented for the tour, grabbed the only pair of jeans I'd packed out of my suitcase, and ducked into the back seat for a quick change of my lower half. The cargo shorts went off, the jeans went on, and that's when the trouble started. I could not for the life of me get my jeans to button closed. I tried multiple times, with all my strength sucking every bit of gut in that I could, and still they were completely unbuttonable. I tried so hard I broke a sweat, and nothing. I got out of the car and stood up, and still nothing. These jeans fit perfectly fine before I began the tour, but after a couple of months of wearing suit pants or my cargo shorts, both of which were much more forgiving, I had managed to outgrow them. I zipped up the jeans as high as they could go, strapped my belt across the unbuttoned front, made sure my shirt covered it, and hoped for the best. I had a drink with my family, enjoyed the view, and never told them about the struggle I'd endured in the car. Later, after saying our goodbyes, I drove to the closest open Walmart and bought the biggest pair of jeans I could find. Thankfully Walmart was ready to cover the oversized masses in a pinch.

This was one of those breaking points that I think all overweight people have in life. A wake-up call that shit just got real. I vowed that I would slim down as soon as I got back to Los Angeles. I think that attempt lasted about three weeks before I started wearing my big-boy pants on a regular basis. After all, they were hella comfortable.

Sometimes we hit snooze too many times on our wake-up call.

Because I expect, and hope, my body will continue to slim down over the next year, I have been reluctant to invest in a new wardrobe. I still have smaller clothes I need to shrink into, but I decided that I will never let myself get as bad as I did and donated the larger sizes. Hopefully, somewhere out there a boat is using my old big-ass Walmart jeans as a sail.

The worst thing about losing this weight is that all my clothes look terrible. Then again, they always looked terrible just tighter.

Well, I did treat myself to a new suit. Also, on Father's Day, my daughter, with help from her mother, surprised me with a great gift: a shirt in a size smaller than what I currently wear, and it fits! I'm not ready to fully update my wardrobe to the smaller size, but it is nice to have more evidence that I have lost weight. A man's got to clean up once in a while.

The Worst Things About Losing One Hundred Pounds

- Most of my clothes are way too big for me.

5

Not That Kind of Bear

As a relatively new author, I pay attention to the reviews people post online. Of course I love it when I see something positive, and most of what I have seen regarding my prior works has been quite positive, but I also appreciate a valid criticism. Nobody wants a negative review, but I get that my work may not be what every reader is expecting. I have seen complaints that a book, written by a comedian psychologist—as indicated on the freaking cover—includes too many jokes or not enough jokes or too much psychology or not enough psychology. You may have thought this book was going to be all about panda bears, and if that was the case, I am sorry to tell you it isn't and ask who is really to blame on that one? How in the world did you make it this far without realizing this is not about pandas?

One criticism of my last book that caught me by surprise was that I came across as slightly fat shaming, which was weird to me, as the only mention of being overweight in my previous works were self-descriptive or self-deprecating jokes. These types of jokes are a staple in any comedian's toolbox, regardless of their body type, and for an overweight comedian they are practically an industry standard. I also made jokes about Sarah cheating on me and not knowing who Alyssa's real father was, but as far as I know nobody accused my last book of slut shaming. Maybe no sluts read the book.

Fat has become political for some reason, and I knew from the beginning that if I were to write a book about losing weight it would trigger some hate from the fat acceptance or body positivity communities. This is definitely not my intention, and I sincerely hope that nothing I write makes anyone feel bad about themselves or other people. I think this should be one of those ideas that should go without saying, but in the current social climate let me be perfectly explicit: nobody should ever be made to feel bad about their physical size or body type.

I grew up fat. I was "husky," as the adults liked to say. I was teased as a child and ostracized as a teenager because of my body weight. Some of that helped me develop my sense of humor and thick skin, but it was still shitty to endure. There are plenty of thin guys who are funny, but fat guys have to tell good jokes.[96] Even as an adult I have been teased maliciously, rejected by women, and passed over for jobs. I have had to either come to terms with or overcome many obstacles in life that would not have been present had I been a smaller size. One of the underlying reasons I have a doctorate is that fewer people would screw me without one. Then

96 I feel like this joke is going to generate some hate.

again, from another perspective I'm not fat; the earth just finds me more attractive than other people.[97]

I am not anti-fat, but I am also not a member of the fat acceptance community. I believe in body positivity; I think everyone should be able to feel comfortable in their own skin and not have to feel shame or humiliation over their physical appearance. Some people look great despite being overweight,[98] but I think I am much more attractive when I am thinner. I am not alone in this opinion either. In the last two weeks I have had three different women tell me they liked my earrings. These are the same ones I've been wearing for years, but I guess they were hard to see around all the extra body fat. If my desire to lose weight was solely motivated by my desire to be more attractive, I would have lost it a long time ago. I'd have visible abs and several other children that I don't know about scattered throughout the world. I also believe that each person should strive to be the best version of themself that they can be. I don't ever want to be content with who I am; there is always room for improvement. Man, if I were thin with a doctorate, I'd be unstoppable on Tinder.

I would never want to be judged solely on my physical appearance, but I would appreciate if it at least opened a few doors for me. Well, there was this one time . . . in college . . . at a summer camp.

Seriously, one summer during college I took a job as a tour guide for a company based in northern California. When we were training or otherwise not on tour, we were allowed to stay at

---

97 Gravity is the force of attraction. This may be the smartest joke in the book; it even went over my editor's head.

98 You may recall that fat distribution, as measured by waist-to-hip ratio, is also an important factor in subjective attractiveness.

a campground in the middle of a small town called Guerneville. About two hours north of San Francisco, Guerneville is a cute town nestled among the redwoods along the Russian River, halfway between Santa Rosa and the ocean. It made for an idyllic camping situation. Had it not been for the fact that while I was there I wasn't being paid, I would have been content to spend my entire summer camping instead of driving vans of tourists to Yosemite National Park.

Guerneville is a tiny town, but it attracts a lot of visitors. After being there for a bit, I learned that it is a popular vacation destination for gay men, in particular a subculture known as "bears." If you are unfamiliar, bears are larger men who are often a bit hairy. Every summer there is an event called Lazy Bear Week, where thousands of large gay men descend onto the streets of town, and I was lucky enough to be camping nearby when it happened that year. At the time, I was not nearly to my peak weight of four hundred pounds—in fact, I probably hadn't yet hit three hundred—but I definitely looked the part as I walked around town. Not being gay, I enjoyed the week simply as a spectator, but damn, did I get some attention. I even had a couple of guys buy me drinks because they thought I was cute.

If I were gay, the title *Of Bears and Weight Loss* would have a much different meaning, and I would definitely be writing it somewhere else.

Gay men who identify as bears and the people who love them are an example of how everyone, despite their physical differences, can be found attractive. There is a market for every body type.

There are people who are specifically attracted to obesity, the so-called "chubby chasers," women who identify as Big Beautiful Women (BBW), and men who identify as Big Handsome Men (BHM). I am not intimately familiar with these communities, but they are evidence that there is a tremendous variety in what physical attributes humans find attractive in others. I had decent luck in my dating life over the years, but the bigger I got, the fewer and further between were the quality relationships. Perhaps I should have signed up for a BHM dating site.

Regardless of whether fat is accepted, tolerated, praised, or even desired, having too much of it increases the risk of a whole lot of health complications down the road. I don't understand how that got so politically charged. Yes, we shouldn't bully people who look different. I want to look better, but my desire to finally lose the weight had everything to do with my health and my desire to spend as much time on this planet with Sarah and Alyssa as I can. I am closer to that goal as I write this, and hopefully I will continue down that path.

FAT TALES

Eating Like Olympians

Earlier this year, I had a short break from my tour schedule and decided to treat my family to a vacation in Puerto Rico. With all our travel, we had accumulated a lot of hotel points, and I used them to book us a resort that I wouldn't normally have paid for out of pocket. It was a nice complex on the south side of the island in Ponce.

When we arrived, we could tell the hotel was preparing for a major event. There were people all over the open-air resort, and everyone seemed very enthusiastic and happy. There was an energy present. Maybe someone leaked that we were going to be there? Yeah, right. Even had we been celebrities, we realized it must have been for some sort of athletic event when we saw displays set up from a few sporting goods manufacturers. If there is one thing my "brand" is not, it's athletic. There were coaches and people in training gear being delivered by the busload. The vibe was really too energetic to have anything to do with a fat comedian and his family.

There was a track event, the Puerto Rico International Athletics Classic, being held nearby and all of its athletes were staying at our hotel. Coincidentally, we arrived on the same day as most of the people involved. I learned that our hotel was hosting several Olympic athletes, including five-time Olympic champion and the fastest woman alive, Elaine Thompson-Herah. Not that I would have recognized any of them, as someone who isn't really into running. I probably haven't run in about thirty years, and the last time was to catch up to an ice cream truck. It just wouldn't stop! My daughter likes to run because, well, she's five, so I asked around a bit and was really lucky to get to introduce her to the fastest woman alive! In our brief encounter, Elaine was very nice and graciously posed for a photo with Alyssa.

The hotel had a nice breakfast buffet, and on the morning after the big event the line was enormous, filled with athletes in top physical condition, a few more regular-looking schlubs, and me, the fat comedian. Standing in line behind so many athletes, I got a kick out of how much food I saw them pile onto their plates. I turned to Sarah and said, "Hey look at that. I eat like an Olympian!" If only I had exercised like one too.

I found out later that Elaine won her race at that event, because of course she did. She is the fastest woman alive.

6

The Right Place at the Right Time

When I realized I was going to be in Montreal to write this book, I was seriously concerned about whether or not I would be able to manage it. To understand why, you should know that it had been over four years since our last visit to our condo. We bought it, then rented it out while we were on tour in the United States, and we were very fortunate that our tenants chose to stay throughout the COVID-19 pandemic. My concern wasn't that I would be unable to write while living in Montreal but that I wouldn't be able to stop myself from eating all of the wonderful foods I had been missing for the last four years. I want my book about weight loss to coincide with some actual weight lost.

Montreal is an amazing city for food. Anthony Bourdain raved about the scene here, and the city boasts a number of world-famous chefs. I assume it all started with the French heritage, because the

French cook some amazing food, and we are surrounded by delicious options wherever we go. French cuisine isn't exactly known for being overly health-conscious, either. As revealed in the movie *Last Holiday*, the secret of life is butter!

Modern Montreal is a melting pot, a fondue if you will, and the foodie scene doesn't just reflect its Parisian roots. Many other cultures have brought their ingredients and specialty dishes to the buffet (a word of French origin, I should point out). There are Jewish delis with their own brand of Montreal smoked meat that has made them famous. I remember reading an interview with actor Brett Kelly who as a child played the chubby kid in *Bad Santa* and spoke about gaining weight for the sequel, *Bad Santa 2* (filmed in Montreal), thirteen years later. He ate a lot of smoked meat sandwiches. He said, "I put on about forty to fifty pounds, and if there's ever a city where you can completely disregard your health, Montreal is probably the place to do it."[99] I love smoked meat, although I have successfully restricted myself to only about two portions of it this summer.

Montreal bagels are a big deal and are awesome. Being from New York originally, I am a bit defensive when it comes to foods that I grew up with, but Montreal-style bagels are an entirely different beast. Yes, technically they are made with similar ingredients as bagels elsewhere and are made into a familiar shape, but they are light and fluffy, with a hint of honey sweetness. They are simply delicious. Like I tell my friends back home, the first time I went to St-Viateur Bagel, I bought a dozen and ate six of them

99 Jesse Johnson, "B.C. Actor Brett Kelly Is Back in *Bad Santa 2* with Billy Bob Thornton" (CBC News, August 16, 2016), https://www.cbc.ca/news/canada/british-columbia/b-c-actor-brett-kelly-is-back-in-bad-santa-2-with-billy-bob-thornton-1.3723669.

immediately while sitting on a bench outside the store. I had never ever eaten six bagels in one sitting before, but these were unlike any other bagels I had tasted. So far this summer, I have successfully avoided a bagel run.

Portuguese chicken is also wildly popular in this city, and one of the greatest restaurants for this dish is a few short blocks from where I am sitting right now. I won't mention it by name because it's already getting too crowded, but wow, I can almost taste it. In our first summer in Montreal, we stayed at an Airbnb down the block and would watch them unload trucks of imported hickory wood from the US. We could smell the smoke from our window and pop our heads out to see how long the line was.

There are wonderful French bakeries, *boulangeries*, literally everywhere, serving up amazing fresh breads and pastries. There is just something so European feeling about taking my daughter and a couple of fresh baguettes to a park bench for a picnic. Luckily Sarah maintains a gluten-free diet, which helps keep my bakery visits to a minimum, and I can't even remember the last time I had pasta since we started dating. Arabic food, dumpling houses, sushi, Brazilian barbeque—all are within reach. From fast food to high-end dining, there are incredible tastes available to satisfy even the most epicurean appetites, and on any budget.

Not that it has anything to do with fine dining, but the popular YouTube show *Epic Meal Time* started here.

I haven't even mentioned the beer. From the iconic Molsons Brewery on the river to the hundreds of microbreweries scattered throughout the city, the people here know how to fuel a party. Thankfully, alcohol has never been my vice of choice.

Clearly, I can't discuss Montreal cuisine without mentioning poutine. Really it should have been the first item on this list, as anyone who has ever visited this city will understand. Poutine, as I shared earlier, is a simple dish invented here that consists of french fries topped with cheese curds and covered in gravy. Cheese fries are common in the States, gravy fries aren't unheard of, and combining all three ingredients isn't that much of a stretch. The thing a lot of Americans don't realize is that in the States that might be an appetizer or a side, but in Canada, that is a meal. And it is super popular. Every restaurant, no matter what type of cuisine or style of service, has poutine on the menu, and many of them will have an entire poutine section with various additional toppings or alternate recipes. My favorite is the General Tso's chicken poutine, which is making me salivate while typing this sentence.

Signs for poutine are everywhere. When I performed comedy in Montreal, I would often talk about how it is so hard to stay healthy here with everyone pushing poutine on you. "Would you like some poutine? It's a Montrealer special recipe!" Sure, I'll try that. "Would you like some more poutine?" Oh man, I don't think I can; I just had a big plate of poutine down the block. "How about if we put some smoked meat on that poutine?" Now you're talking! "How about some Portuguese chicken on the poutine?" Oh man, I'm sure I can find some room somewhere—let me shuffle around some inner organs. "How about some maple syrup poutine for dessert?" What the hell; when in Rome, right? I hear you guys have free health care.

And then there is the syrup. Maple syrup is so incredibly popular here that they advertise it on the national flag. They named

Toronto's hockey team after it. I love maple syrup and, unfortunately for a guy trying to drop some weight, it is ubiquitous here. In winter, and at tourist spots year-round, they serve a maple taffy that is distilled syrup poured over snow until it hardens and is then rolled onto a stick. Cold maple syrup on a stick! Whoever started that should get a damn Nobel Prize. It's not just syrup, either. Maple flavoring seems to add a special flavor, and calories, to anything and everything. There are traditional sugar shacks, or *cabanes à sucre*, serving up all sorts of maple goodies, that are sprinkled all over the region and are almost as alluring as a good waist-to-hip ratio. I think maple is my favorite way to consume sugar, and I particularly love it in my coffee.

Speaking of sugar, this reminds me of something else about Montreal that excites me more than it should: caramel spread. This is a popular staple used on toast, the same as you might use jelly, honey, or marmalade. I first learned of its existence the morning after a hotel stay when I went down to the lobby to take advantage of the free breakfast. The container caught my attention. What is this? Caramel made to spread on toast? That is insane, and deliciously awesome! I'll be honest—it doesn't seem much different from caramel sauce packaged for ice cream, so of course it tastes great on toast. It's freaking caramel! I'm no connoisseur, but I love the stuff. Maybe it's based on products available in France, but the main brand here is made just outside of Montreal.

Canada also allows for the consumption of many foods that are unavailable in the United States, like horse meat and seal. Since I know you are curious, I did end up cooking my seal burgers, and they were very tasty. You can really taste the flipper! Sarah liked it too, but I couldn't convince our daughter to try them with us.

So yeah, it may seem like I am in the wrong place to write a weight loss book, but given all of the various temptations I am surrounded with, I have been doing surprisingly well. I have taken my daughter to get baguettes a few times and indulged in some maple products throughout the last two months; however, I have only had poutine twice, and for one of those occasions I was introducing some American friends to the joys of Montreal eating.[100] I have yet to visit my favorite Portuguese chicken place, and although I've walked by the St-Viateur Bagel shop a few times, I haven't been in once.

What is making the difference this time is that we have a kitchen. We are staying in our home for the first time since we bought it, not some rental or hotel, and we aren't here as tourists. We get to buy groceries, stock a pantry, and cook for ourselves. You know, like normal people. We were tourists for all of our prior visits, and part of the excitement of travel is exploring new foods and learning about a culture by the way it eats. Playing house for the summer has kept us from partaking in virtually all of the goodies I listed. Although I will admit we have indulged a few times (probably more than we should have), having a kitchen has helped make it a relatively healthy stay. That, and my strong desire to continue losing my extra weight and keep that promise to Alyssa.

You know what else Montreal has? Some great farmers markets located in convenient spots all over the city. Our favorite is the Jean Talon, an open-air market full of farm-fresh produce and other items from local vendors. Sure, there isn't anything wrong

100 They hadn't yet had a chance to read this book, given that I am still in the process of writing it.

with regular grocery stores, but going to a market is an event. It isn't just shopping; it's recreation. Not only is it a joy to visit, but we always come home with lots of healthy foods to stock our fridge.

There is also an abundance of vegetarian restaurants here, serving up food for diet-conscious consumers, and most places have plenty of vegetarian or low-calorie options. Montreal has some good eating, but it isn't difficult to eat healthy here.

That addresses the eating, but what about the exercise?

At the entrance to Chinatown there is a paifang (an ornate gateway) with an inscription that translates to "A splendid environment fosters a great people."[101] I think a version of this would make a great slogan for the entire city. Although it is a city that seems to offer a little of everything when it comes to vice, at the same time it helps to foster a healthy lifestyle for those who care about that sort of thing.

One of the things that Sarah and I fell in love with about Montreal is how extremely walkable it is, and we walk everywhere. On most days, I easily get my steps in just by going about my business.[102] Part of that is our location. We are within a fifteen-minute walk to the major festival areas, twenty minutes to downtown, thirty to the old port historic area, twenty to either La Fontaine Park (Parc La Fontaine) or the base of Mount Royal, and most days we can get our exercise by wandering around the neighborhood. Unless we are stocking up, we will walk to a corner grocery store, called a *dépanneur* here, or to a larger supermarket. Bars,

---

101 According to Alan Hustak and Johanne Norchet, *Montréal Then and Now* (San Diego, CA: Thunder Bay Press, 2006).

102 Unfortunately, writing requires a lot of sitting with a computer, but even when the inspiration hits and the ideas keep flowing, I try to get out and stretch my legs for at least an hour a day.

theaters, and comedy venues are usually within walking distance. Having a five-year-old's legs, Alyssa uses her scooter to traverse the city with us when she's not sprouting caterpillars. Granted we live in a central area, but even the neighborhoods in the outskirts have their business districts and pedestrian-friendly areas.

A lot of Montreal's walkability is a function of the existing infrastructure and whatever urban planning led to the current conditions, but as I mentioned, the city attempts to foster a healthy lifestyle. Over the summer many streets that are normally busy with car traffic are designated as pedestrian-only zones, making them perfect places to walk around and explore. This not only makes walking, and therefore exercise, more desirable, but it also discourages driving. We only drive when we have big shopping to do, or need to leave town for a bit, but otherwise our car sits there parked, enjoying the break from its normal touring gig.

Bicycle use is encouraged, and there are bike lanes on all the major thoroughfares. We did not bring our bikes up for this stay, but the city has its own bike-sharing system (it was actually the first large-scale one in North America), and I have found them to be super convenient. I haven't ridden much, but it seems that car traffic is fairly respectful to bike riders, and speaking of traffic . . .

When you're driving or biking in Montreal, and only in Montreal, it is always against the law to make a right turn at a red light. Montreal is the last city in North America to have this restriction city-wide, and I never fully understood why it does, but evidently the primary argument in favor of maintaining this law is pedestrian safety. They want you to walk in Montreal and feel safe while doing it. So get off your butt and take a walk.

In many ways, Montreal reminds me of Europe. Most older cities with well-developed cores are highly walkable. I have lived in a bunch of cities in the United States, including New York City, Philadelphia, New Orleans, and San Francisco. Those cities are also highly walkable in their cores, and I love them for it. But in most American cities, and metro areas, walkability tends to break down the farther from downtown you travel. A lot of American cities encourage car dependence in just a few blocks. Unless Europe has radically changed since my last visit three years ago, that isn't the case there. Obviously, the city cores in Europe have a bit of a historical head start over their American counterparts, but as a casual observer it seemed to me that they have grown differently in the time since cars have existed.

Come to think of it, Sarah and I saw very few drive-through restaurants in Europe. They were there, but they're not nearly as ubiquitous as in the United States. We were convinced that Switzerland didn't even allow them, as we entered in Geneva and drove all over the country without seeing one until we finally passed one days later near Zurich. By the way, if you really want an awkward tourist experience, try driving an English car (driver on the right side) through a European McDonald's drive-through without someone sitting in the passenger seat to assist with the order.

I have known many people who seem to romanticize Europe's public transportation use and how much people walk or bike to get around, but trust me, I am not one of those people. Plenty of people drive in Europe. Traffic in some cities is ridiculous. Driving in downtown London is a massive pain in the arse (that's for you,

England), and I challenge you to find a more thrilling carnival ride than circling the Arc de Triomphe in Paris. Europe is not the carless utopia that some Americans imagine it to be, and there is plenty of traffic. However, compared to traffic in most cities in the United States, it seems that a larger portion of that traffic is on the sidewalks, where people are moving their bodies to get around. Just like in Montreal.

Getting Those Last Few Steps In

Walking really is my favorite form of exercise. It is easy and almost anyone can do it. I've been doing it since I was about a year old, and I like to think I am somewhat of an expert on it. To date I've walked on four continents. Running, on the other hand, is a skill I have yet to master. Yet, ironically, I know how to dance the Running Man.

Walking for the sole purpose of getting exercise does get boring for me. I can't do a treadmill. This is why I have always preferred to live in walkable cities and neighborhoods; just going about my business takes the focus off the exercise and puts it onto the activity or objective. I'm not taking a walk just to get some arbitrary number of steps in; I'm walking to check out a comedy show or taking a photographic tour of street art. In other words,

I'm going somewhere. I'm doing something. I distract my brain from the exercise by focusing on some more interesting activity that it enjoys. I will walk around Old Montreal or Le Plateau for hours. I will walk pretty much nonstop in New Orleans during Mardi Gras. If I put myself in a stimulating enough environment, and load up with enough strands of plastic beads, I can walk indefinitely.

I taught my daughter to walk in Florida, and she's a master walker. She also likes to run, and I promised her a long time ago that someday Daddy is going to run with her. Now that she has met the fastest woman alive, that may pose more of a challenge for me in the future.

Of course, there are times when I get lazy. Even in this environment of central Montreal, there are moments when I don't feel like putting forth the effort to walk a few blocks to get something to eat. However, even my laziness has its limits.

I have never used a food delivery app like Uber Eats, Grubhub, DoorDash, LazyMan, or Fuzed2thecouch. Don't get me wrong, I'm not trying to claim some faux superiority like the people who smugly say things like "I don't even own a television." I use plenty of apps, and I have ordered plenty of food for delivery, as long as that food is pizza and it's delivered in thirty minutes or less. My main reason for not using these delivery apps is that I've never been so hungry (or high) that I would be willing to pay a few extra bucks for someone else to make my run to Taco Bell, pick up my bean burrito with the extra red sauce, and bring it to me. At least with the pizza guys, the delivery staff is already in the restaurant. Fast food is caloric enough, but in the old days you had to actually go out in public and exert a little energy if you wanted to overeat. Then came the drive-through, which eliminated all the exercise we would get walking between our car and the restaurant, allowing the laziest among us to purchase and dine without ever leaving the comfort of our driver's seat. Then came the delivery apps, removing the need to walk from our couch to our car and the last bit of exercise we had left if we wanted to stuff our face full of french fries. If there was some service that would tackle that remaining door-to-mouth distance, I'm sure there would be a market for it.

I don't think that everyone who uses these apps is lazy, or even that laziness is the primary motivator for their use. My point is that as great as these modern conveniences are, they reduce our need to engage in physical activity. Thanks to Amazon, many of us don't even get the benefit of walking through a mall to go shopping anymore. On the rare occasion I find myself inside a mall or a big department store, I am overcome with feelings of nostalgia. "Oh wow, this is how we used to do things in the old days!" For the past several years, and understandably throughout the pandemic, delivery services have been extremely helpful and in turn have become very popular. However, I would still rather use my feet and get those last few steps in as long as I am able.

But wait, you mean I can order food from my favorite restaurant and I don't even have to put on pants? There may be something to this.

SPEAKING OF EUROPE

German Comedian Thomas Nicolai

From the ages of eight to twelve I lived in Frankfurt, Germany. It was my first time leaving my home country, and I remember not having a concept of what that meant. In contrast, my daughter is five and she has already visited eleven countries with hopefully more in the near future.

Because I was so young, I don't have strong memories of my time in Germany, but I do recall noticing that I couldn't understand what most people were saying when we got off the airplane. Eventually, I would learn some of the language, enough to have German-speaking friends and later have it interfere with my attempts to learn Spanish in college.

I never went back to Germany, or any of Europe, until almost forty years later. Therefore, my impression of the European lifestyle may not be all that accurate. For this I decided to consult another expert.

The German version of my book *The Art of Taking It Easy* was recorded as an audiobook read by the well-known German comedian and voice artist Thomas Nicolai. I thought, who better to provide me with some insight on the health-related behaviors of Europe?

Brian: Could you first tell my readers a little about yourself and career?

Thomas: I was born in Leipzig, which is in the former German Democratic Republic,[103] in 1963. My father was a jazz musician and played the piano. My mother came from a large family of artists. Even as a child, I had a lot to do with artists and other weirdos. That shaped me. And pretty early on, I thought that's what I wanted to do.

I began studying at the East Berlin Drama School in 1987. I was an actor with a diploma and had my first engagement at the GRIPS Theater, a children and youth theater in Berlin. During this time I was already playing in small clubs and doing comedy. I sang funny songs with a jazz guitarist. That went down great from the beginning. I thought that was OK, because I was extremely convinced of myself.

In the mid-nineties, I left theater and since then I've made a living out of making people laugh. The comedy and stand-up scene in Germany was still very young [when I started]. There were already a few stars, but they shared the halls among themselves in the German-speaking countries. I wrote my programs and went on tour with them. This time with a keyboard player who could realize my crazy ideas of song parodies better than my guitarist at that time.

My specialties are song parodies and impressions of weird guys. It didn't take long before the first TV appearances followed. I even had my own personality show on German television (for a short time) and a record contract with Sony. One could think I

103 East Germany.

had made it, that I was a superstar.

Admittedly, sometimes I also felt like that. But I never really had a big breakthrough. I think my humor is not mainstream enough. I like it a little more offbeat. Maybe it has to do with the fact that I come from the theater. By the way, the cliché that Germans don't have a sense of humor is not true at all. Today we have a very lively and large comedy scene in Germany.

And then COVID-19 came along. I had already worked a lot as a voice actor for dubbing, commercials, and radio plays. I've been recording audiobooks for over three years now. That saved me financially during the pandemic. And as the pandemic is not over yet, it will save me in the next months (and years?) as well.

Brian: For a guy approaching sixty, you seem to keep yourself in pretty good shape. Have you ever struggled managing body weight?

Thomas: Until I turned thirty, I thought it didn't matter what I ate, when I ate, and especially how much I ate. I ate and drank and had fun. Going to the pub and partying and boozing. No problem. Things started to change in my mid-thirties at the latest. Not abruptly, but noticeably.

From the age of forty at the latest, you have to start living more consciously and also decide whether you want to continue living the way you have been. Can I go on living like this, do I want to go on living like this, and can I afford to go on living like this? Am I doing my body any good by continuing to live this way?

I'm an actor and comedian, and I work a lot with my body and my voice. My body is my house, and my body is my tool. I have to take care of it; otherwise it will eventually break and I won't be able to use it. At my live shows I sing for two hours, songs that range from classical to heavy metal, and I jump across the stage. I also talk without taking a breath, dress up all the time, and have to show that I'm having an incredible amount of fun (which I am), and act like it doesn't strain me at all, so that the audience thinks that the guy is a real professional. But how am I supposed to do that when I'm out of breath, my joints hurt, and I have back pain?

Because I love my job, there was no other answer for me: I had to change something. Not radically, just by living a little more consciously. The result of my path has proven itself.

But one thing is clear: nothing happens on its own without doing something. There is a fundamental attitude to it that starts in the head. The reward is a body that works and doesn't hurt you permanently.

Brian: How do you manage to stay in shape?

Thomas: I started to eat more consciously. It is clear that eating is a lot of fun and that good food is an absolute happiness maker. But I noticed that I very often ate indiscriminately, and if it tasted good, I ate quickly, very quickly. Yes, I think I was in the top five of the world's fastest eaters. I tried to balance that with sports, but to be honest, I was the most unathletic person ever until then. It didn't interest me. And if I'm honest, it still doesn't interest me to this day. For a short time I joined a fitness center, but that stressed me out. All around me were super ambitious guys pumping up their muscles. I felt like a loser twice. Unathletic and pale, with strings instead of muscles. Embarrassing. I canceled my membership to the fitness center.

Fortunately, a short time later I started jogging. That's exactly my thing. I can do it alone, without time pressure, for as long as I want. If I can manage, I run three times a week, forty-five minutes each time. Put some good music or a podcast in my ears and it's perfect.

But, and this is the most important thing, I actually pay attention to my diet. Better food, less sweets, less alcohol, enough sleep, less stress, happier living. Simply more enjoyment and not stuffing so much into myself.

The body is an incredibly great organism because it constantly gives us signals. If you exercise too much, it hurts you right away, and if you are full, your body will tell you that too.

Because food tastes so damn delicious, we keep ignoring these signs and thinking to ourselves, *No, don't stop. I'm still hungry. Please have another huge serving of spaghetti Bolognese. And another hamburger. And eight scoops of ice cream and . . . wait, my pants are stretching?*

One problem is snacking on sweets. Imagine sitting in front of the TV and watching a cool Netflix series while stuffing chocolate, chips, or popcorn down your throat. *Oops, I already ate the second bag? I'll see if there's anything sweet or salty left in the apartment. If necessary, I'll eat some cheese from the fridge. That tastes good too. After all, I still have two episodes to watch. It's so exciting. And I can't watch TV without snacking. Oh, can I have another large beer?*

It's a bad habit, but one that can be broken. I can only snack on what's there. If the cupboard in the living room is so full of sweets and salty treats that you can't get the door shut, then everyone will say, "Well, come on, we have to change that. Bring on the sweets."

But if there's very little in the cupboard, my consumption is limited. I can only eat what's there.

Do I want to live like an ascetic? Do I want to become a health apostle and constantly get on the nerves of others and lecture those around me? I don't think anyone wants that. But I say from my own experience, this snacking in front of the TV is a senseless and above all completely thoughtless consumption of many calories that we actually do not need.

Consciously snacking and enjoying is better and healthier.

Of course, you can and should have sweets [and salty snacks] in the house, but it doesn't have to be ten bars of chocolate and twenty bags of chips. Finding the right balance is the trick.

I don't think an ascetic life is the right path for me. I'm far too much of a pleasure seeker for that. I love my life. It's nice to celebrate with friends and to eat and drink. That is part of life.

My way is to try to live more consciously. I don't do without anything. I do eat and drink everything—but everything in moderation, and I succeed better than I can describe. For me it's all about the right balance.

What also helps me is the so-called interval fasting according to the 18:6 principle. You don't eat anything for eighteen hours, then you have a window of six hours when you can eat. I admit that this sounds very German and not feasible for many people.

People who have to work hard physically cannot implement this interval. The body simply needs power for physically demanding jobs. I, however, am a freelance comedian and can do it with ease. I've already been able to get rid of many an annoying kilo this way.

Brian: Do you think Germany has an obesity epidemic?

Thomas: I am not a scientist, doctor, psychologist, or sociologist. I can only describe what I see. And I see a lot of fat people in Germany. I know that doctors in Germany are talking about an obesity epidemic. I think it's exaggerated, but then I'm not an expert.

What surprises me, however, is that here in Germany, on the one hand we have a very high level of education on the subject of "healthy eating" and many also live by it, while others are not interested at all.

Brian: I am currently in Montreal, surrounded by french fry pushers, maple syrup sellers, and the constant smell of French baked goods. Is German food healthy?

Thomas: Absolutely not. German food consists of meat, fat, lots of cream, and potatoes. Maybe sometimes vegetables (but who likes to eat vegetables voluntarily?). And the Germans like to eat a lot.

Add to that a large beer and a German is the happiest person in the world.

German cuisine is great and there are many ingenious dishes that taste incredibly good, but the ingredients are not so healthy. But that's the way it is with food: the things that taste the best are not always the healthiest. If you know that and accept it, you're already a big step further in the state of knowledge.

I remember a TV show I was invited on. It was a cooking show where the celebrities were supposed to cook. I had chosen meatloaf with mashed potatoes as my dish. On the day of the taping, I met with my chef in the afternoon and he prepared me and gave me some tips for my dish.

He asked me about the ingredients for my mashed potatoes. I said, "I boil the potatoes, drain the water, and add a spoonful of butter and a little milk, salt, and nutmeg."

"That's all?" he asked.

"Yes," I confirmed.

"No," he said, "you have to put in a lot of crème fraîche. Otherwise Calli won't eat it." Calli's real name is Reiner Calmund, and he is a very popular former soccer manager who has become known primarily for his oversized fat belly, and he was sitting on the jury.

When the show came on in the evening, I followed my professional chef's tip and added a good amount of crème fraîche to the mashed potatoes. And Calli was thrilled.

"These are the best mashed potatoes I've ever had in my life." With these words, he reached next to him to the neighboring jury colleague and ate her mashed potatoes too.

Why? Crème fraîche is a flavor enhancer. You want more and more of it, and you even end up licking the plate, it's that delicious. Granted, with it the dish really does taste a lot better. But it also has calories without end.

Brian: I lived in Germany as a child, and from what I remember—and my impressions as an adult tourist—there is a great deal of emphasis on physical activity compared to the United States. For example, walking as a means to get around seemed a lot more common. I remember the bike trails all over Frankfurt, and I still have my old Volksmarch walking stick with several shields.[104] Do

---

104 Volksmarching is a form of noncompetitive hiking. I remember there being fairly regular events for it, and at the end we would be rewarded with a small shield-shaped badge to attach to our walking stick.

you think this is an accurate assessment?

Thomas: Yes, a lot of sport is actually being done in Germany. Fitness studios are springing up like mushrooms, and more and more people, old and young, want to look healthy and strong.

It's normal to take care of your body and keep moving. This includes taking walks. In Germany they say, "You snooze, you rust."

Is there a difference between Europe and America concerning this problem? I don't know enough about it. But I remember doing a little trip through the United States many years ago and I was first amazed at the slim New Yorkers, but then in the Midwest I was amazed at the very fat people.[105] To be honest, I had never seen anything like that before and didn't know that such a thing was even possible, that the human organism and bones could manage it.

But I also found the supermarkets remarkable. They were incredibly large and seemed to have no end. And the huge packages of food were enough to feed a whole village.

I also found it strange that the fast food restaurants were full, but at the Chinese or Italian restaurant there was no problem to find a table. For me, it was a topsy-turvy world.

I remember eating a hamburger in Dallas that was three times as big as the ones in Germany and seemed to consist only of fat. When I ate that monster, I felt really bad.

Brian: What about Americans you see in Germany? Are there any health-related behaviors you see more from American tourists as opposed to those from locals or tourists from other countries?

---

105 Whenever I have toured in that region, I have gotten a lot of use out of this introductory joke: "I love being in the Midwest. Out here, nobody knows I'm fat."

Thomas: I'm sorry, there's not much I can say about that. Of course, there is the cliché of the fat and loud American. But I've also met many Americans who are very smart and open-minded.

Berlin is a hotspot. Some days I have the impression that the whole world is in this city right now. I find that very comforting.

We humans have the chance to grow together. I think that's very beautiful. And when I look at what I eat now, I have the feeling that we've already come a long way.

Brian: While I have you, I have to ask: What's the deal with David Hasselhoff?

Thomas: Ha ha! That's a wonderful question. I think everyone here loves David Hasselhoff because no one really takes him seriously. And I don't think he takes himself that seriously either.

He became immortal when he stood on the Berlin Wall in 1989 and sang the song "Looking for Freedom." He was wearing a glitter jacket with glow bulbs. It was so crazy, and so totally surreal, that all Germans took him to their hearts.

The Hoff is its own planet with its own orbit. People like that don't get built anymore. The Hoff is America totally, but somehow it also belongs to Germany.

FAT TALES

The Adventures of Daddy Pig

I wrote my previous book while living in Denver, over the last three months of 2018. Sarah had taken a short-term therapy contract at a clinic there, and I had a few months off from my tour schedule. We found a nice furnished rental that served our needs. It even had a fireplace, which came in handy on the days that Colorado winter weather was a bit too wintery.

The one major downside was that it had a limited selection of TV channels. Sarah was working outside of the home, and I was writing a book while taking care of our daughter. Alyssa was about one and a half at the time, which meant that, as a stay-at-home dad, if I was going to get any writing done, I needed to find some cartoons on that TV. Fortunately, there was one channel that kept her attention although I had never heard of any of the shows. One of them was a simple cartoon about a family of British pigs called *Peppa Pig*. The show centered on a little girl pig named Peppa; her brother, George; and her parents, Mummy Pig and Daddy Pig, who were named with such a lack of creativity I am surprised I wasn't one of the writers. The art was simple and the character details were minimal. Each of the parents was drawn with some basic defining features: Mummy Pig had eyelashes and Daddy Pig had facial hair, wore glasses, and sported a big round tummy.

Each episode seemed to involve the most mundane, boring tasks. They would make pancakes, they would watch a TV show about a potato, and they would feed ducks. Yay, excitement. At first I didn't see the appeal, but then again I am outside of the show's target demographic by a few years. It was nice enough, though, and the stories were sweet and family-oriented, but most importantly my daughter was super engaged. Over the course of those three months, she became whatever their fans are called. Peppies? Peppaheads? Bacon lovers?

I could never have predicted how much this little show would influence our lives for the next couple of years.

Let me fill in some back story first. Sarah and I orginally came to Montreal the summer before our daughter was born. However, it was not our planned destination for that trip. After talking to many American comedians about how well received they were overseas, I had been wanting to check out the London comedy scene for a while. Sarah had always wanted to go to England as well, so we thought we would hop across the Atlantic for the summer and check it out. We waited a little too long to book our flights, and when we finally sat down to buy some tickets, prices were ridiculous. Still having the desire to leave the United States for a bit, we started discussing options and I mentioned Canada, another country Sarah had not yet been to. We looked at our calendar, made some arrangements, and soon were heading north to spend the summer exploring the Trans-Canada Highway, from Montreal to Vancouver and up to the Yukon. Had tickets to London been cheaper, or had we not waited so long to buy them, our lives would be radically different right now. In an alternate universe, there is a version of me sitting in a flat in the South Bank of London, writing a book on how to lose weight while trying not to indulge in all the fish and chips at the pubs.

When Sarah's contract in Denver came to an end, I delivered my manuscript to my publisher and we left Colorado to go back on tour. This was now 2019, and we had every intention of finally making it to England that summer. We had renters living in our Montreal home and were itching to make good on a trip we'd promised ourselves, so we made damn sure that we bought our tickets well in advance. Shortly after my last gig, Sarah, Alyssa, and I boarded a plane in Dallas and headed to London to spend a month on the road in Europe.

Almost immediately after passing through customs, we were bombarded with reminders that *Peppa Pig* is an English show. Souvenir shops stocked lots of Peppa toys, something we hadn't seen a lot of back home (yet),[106] and images of the simply drawn pig, which basically looks like a pink whistle with eyes, were ubiquitous. When we checked into our hotel, which was located in an area my friend London-based comedian Julius Howe described as "a bit stabby,"[107] to my daughter's delight, *Peppa Pig* was on multiple TV channels.

After spending a couple days exploring London, Sarah and I learned that there is a *Peppa Pig* theme park in Hampshire that was about two hours away. Without telling Alyssa, we checked out of our hotel on the last morning, hopped in the car, and set out for

106 Lately it seems as if *Peppa Pig* merchandise has made it to the market in the United States in a big way.

107 Stabbings do seem to make headlines there, but not once did it feel like an unsafe neighborhood. Besides, in America, our neighborhoods have guns.

Peppa Pig World. This was not how I originally envisioned I would spend my time in England, but I reasoned that it was Alyssa's trip too and she needed some special experiences of her own.

Peppa must have been on her mind that morning because as I was driving, in her high-pitched two-year-old voice, we heard her say, "I'm Peppa Pig!" She pointed at Sarah, "Mommy Pig!" and then to me, "and you are Daddy Pig!"

I joked to Sarah, "Did she call me fat? Things just got real!"

I'll admit, the resemblance is there. I wear glasses, I usually have facial hair, and there is no denying I carry a version of Daddy's big tummy, but I knew that was not what she meant. For the first time since we met, she was making an analogy and recognizing the similarities between the Pig family and our own. I was happy to note this stage in her development. I turned to look back at her and smile, knowing she was going to love where we were taking her that day.

She wasn't the only one.

I must say it was pretty great. All of the rides were themed from the show and perfectly age appropriate and safe. Alyssa went on all of them. We were able to do some as a family, such as a boat ride and a train ride, and Sarah and I alternated when on the two-seaters. We saw the duck pond, toured the family's house, and even splashed around a bit in muddy puddles like they do on the show. The park was reasonably priced, and so were the food options (the café was named after Daddy Pig, naturally). However, the constant theme song playing in the background was enough to drive any adult nuts, and I feared for my sanity. I swore if any other kids called me "Daddy Pig," I was going to start charging for photos.

Alyssa had a blast. She even got a chance to meet Peppa Pig, live and in person. On the way out we picked up a few souvenirs for her.

Before I became a parent, I would have been cracking jokes all over this wholesome scene, but the last two years with Alyssa had me pretty subdued.

Peppa Pig World is actually a themed section of a larger park, Paultons Park, but it is clearly their main attraction. We were pleased to discover that the entire park was geared toward younger children. There were a lot of grassy spaces and everything was clean, and families more prepared than ours brought picnic baskets and treated themselves to a nice day. I don't think I've ever seen another theme park that would allow that.

When we were finished in the Peppa Pig section, we explored a little more of the rest of Paultons Park and found a really cool rollercoaster, which Alyssa wanted to ride. She specifically wanted me to ride it with her and got very excited about it. I love a good roller coaster and Sarah was happy to sit this one out, so she found a nearby bench. Alyssa and I got in the line, which didn't seem that long, and after about twenty minutes it was our turn to board. We hopped onto the ride and soon discovered that Daddy Pig's big tummy was too big to close the safety harness.

I tried to suck it in, I shifted my fat in every direction, but it wasn't going to work. I was a little embarrassed that I was delaying the ride for everyone else, so I offered to get off, which resulted in a very disappointed daughter. The ride operators wouldn't let Alyssa ride by herself and she started to cry. Just then I spotted Sarah, who was sitting nearby, and asked her to hurry in and swap places with me. She charged into action, skipping past the line, and quickly took my spot in the ride next to Alyssa.

At least Alyssa got to ride it with one of her parents.

When we went to England, I had already been losing weight, but fat was still very much a presence in my life. I had been denied seats on carnival rides before, but this was the first time my size got in the way of enjoying something with my daughter and nearly cost her the experience as well. It was another reminder that no matter how difficult the struggle, I needed to stay on the journey.

When I made a promise to my daughter that I would get healthier, I was thinking about the impact being fat had on my health, but it also limits opportunities and activities. Getting healthier not only means I might be there with her as she grows up but that I can do more and share more with her. Although, now at five, she is telling me not to lose the rest of my weight because I "won't look as good skinny." She is so sweet, but I owe it to her not to honor that request.

When we left the park, we settled into a hotel in Southampton and went out for dinner at a nearby kebab house. Outside the restaurant was a sandwich board sign that read, "Fat people are harder to kidnap. Stay safe!"

So there's at least one bright side to all of this.

The next day we got up and drove to Stonehenge and Oxford before heading toward the English Channel and the ferry to the rest of Europe. We toured around France from Calais through Amiens, Paris (that city Peppa Pig went to!), Lyon, and into the

Alps to visit some friends living in Courchevel.[108] We then went through Switzerland, up the western side of Germany (including my first return to Frankfurt), and over to the Netherlands and Belgium, before finishing the loop and heading back to London.

For the entire trip, Alyssa had been watching *Peppa Pig* first thing in the morning and before going to bed. She had a Peppa Pig doll, which she carried to most places, and loved her new *Peppa Pig* T-shirts and sunglasses. On our last day in England, Sarah and I decided that instead of spending another day exploring London, we would end the month by returning to Peppa Pig World. It turned out to be the best decision we could have made.

For several months after returning to the States, when people asked my daughter what her name was, she always replied, "Peppa."

I don't know how old my daughter was when she first understood that I was overweight, but I do remember one day we were walking and she pointed out another person with a weight problem: "Look, Daddy, that person is your type of person." It took me a moment to understand what she meant, but she was starting to recognize that human beings come in all sorts of shapes. She loves me, and has never taken issue with my weight nor how it has interfered with our lives so far, and I never want her to have to.

108 Our friends work at a ski resort where one of them is a chef. They treated us to some amazing homemade cuisine that was definitely not on the diet. One evening, we had a raclette, a local meal in the Alps. The one they served us was made with cheese, potatoes, and ham. It was amazing. My friend Alex reminded me that I described the sensation of eating it as feeling like I was swimming in grease after having an orgy of cheese.

7

Check Out This Bunch of Losers

This week the Just for Laughs Comedy Festival is going on in Montreal for its first year back since the beginning of the pandemic. You have probably heard of it, but for the uninitiated, it is the largest comedy festival in the world. For audiences, the main draws are the big shows. The festival gets some of the top comedic talents in the world, and for a solid week this city is crawling with celebrity comedians. For us lower-tier comedians who aren't booked to perform, the draw is an opportunity to meet and learn from those who have experienced greater success in the industry. As a comedy fan as well as a performer, I fall a bit into both of those categories, but this year I am sitting out to write this thing you are currently holding.

Because I am missing out on the festival, I thought it would be interesting to reach out to comedians who have lost significant weight. As I mentioned earlier, there is no shortage of overweight comedians in the world. However, a lot of them have made some positive changes in their lives. Also, having gained back a little before arriving in Montreal, I find just discussing weight loss with other people and hearing their stories to be very inspirational.

Comedian Mark Schiff Lost Fifty Pounds After Some Inspiration from Jerry Seinfeld

When I first told a handful of people about my intention to write this book, a few made suggestions of other comedians that I should talk with. One name that came up a couple of times was Mark Schiff. He's not quite a household name, but trust me, this guy is well known in the entertainment community. He started performing stand-up comedy in New York City in the late seventies. His "freshman class" included some names you may recognize, like Gilbert Gottfried, Paul Reiser, Larry Miller, George Wallace, and his good friend that he has been touring with for over twenty years, Jerry Seinfeld.

New York is, and always has been, a breeding ground for the performing arts, and I know it may not seem like it sometimes, but comedy is an art. Growing up there, Mark knew he wanted to do stand-up when he was twelve years old, when his parents took him to see Rodney Dangerfield. He said, "That's it. I know what I want to do for a living," and never looked back. I am from New York as well and also list Rodney Dangerfield as one of my early inspirations (I still have a very worn cassette copy of *Rappin' Rodney* in storage), but when I was coming of age in rural Texas during the late eighties, it was a lot less obvious how to break into that world. In New York, Mark just started performing everywhere he could. When comedy clubs started opening up in the eighties, he could do five sets a night and began headlining because the clubs were so new that competition was sparse. In comedy, it seems that environment counts for a lot.

Mark has been working consistently for over fifty years. He has appeared on the *Tonight Show* with Johnny Carson and Jay Leno, *Late Night with David Letterman*, and *An Evening at the Improv*, and he's written for TV shows starring the likes of Roseanne Barr and Jeff Foxworthy. To put it mildly, we clearly run in different circles. We have never met in person, but thankfully, a mutual friend was able to put us in contact, and Mark, who has also written a book about his career,[109] was gracious enough to talk to me.

Brian: You've had an incredible career in comedy and broadcasting, and now I understand that you've lost a significant amount of weight?

Mark: Fifty pounds! It took me a year to lose it, and I've had it off for ten years.

109 Mark Schiff, *Why Not? Lessons on Comedy, Courage, and Chutzpah* (New York: Apollo Publishers, 2022).

Brian: Were you always heavy growing up?

Mark: No, I was like a Thanksgiving Day balloon. I would blow up once in a while and then let the air out.

I found a picture of myself the other day from when I met Mickey Mantle, the great Yankees baseball player. I was as thin as a rail thirtysomething years ago, and then I really pudged up.

I know some of you hundred pounders think we're teetotalers compared to you, but fifty pounds is a lot of weight, and to keep it off is miserable.

Brian: Yeah, it's tough. I've lost a hundred, but in the course of losing that I probably gained and dropped the same ten or twenty pounds repeatedly over that entire span, and I've still got a bit to go. So you were going up and down for a while, and then you decided to take charge, lose it, and keep it off. Was there a breaking point that made you want to make that change in your life?

Mark: It was a slow progression of giving up bad habits. I'm an alcoholic, so I drank for many years, and I quit that on November 18, 1984. That was the first step: quit the drinking. I was a blackout drinker. Let's say I would go on the road with you for two weeks. We'd hit some club and then I would see you back in town. I wouldn't even remember going on the road with you.

I quit the drinking and then I started ballooning up a little, because when you quit one thing, something else rears its head when you have an addictive personality, and that's me.

I was a periodic exerciser. One day when I was fat, fifty pounds up, I was walking with Seinfeld, and there's a guy with a walker, an old guy. I'll never forget this. Seinfeld said to me, "You see that guy? You don't ever have to be that guy if you don't want to."

And the next day I started exercising and got a grip on myself.

I became a vegetarian thirty-two years ago. That didn't keep the weight off, because you can eat pizza and french fries and drink Coke as a vegetarian. Eventually I became a vegan, which I am now. It's not necessary to lose weight and keep it off, but I find it a healthier alternative.

I have this special thing that I do. By myself, I'm basically helpless. I'm an out-of-control guy, so I started a group with two other guys, and we check in with each other every day. I'll call my friend Bernie in New York and go, "I'm done with my exercise for today." We're committed to exercising seven days a week, which means you probably do six. I call him every day, and I call somebody else. I go, "I'm done exercising." Then I give him a list of foods I don't eat anymore. "No pizza, pasta, bread, frozen yogurt, chips, dips, desserts, fried stuff, licorice, overeating, sugar, sugar substitutes, popcorn, or oil." That's today's list. I don't want to have any of those ever again. All of them do me in. I can't stop eating chips when I eat them. I can't stop eating doughnuts when I eat them. I can't stop drinking soda when I drink it. I can't stop eating pancakes. All of it, if they're in front of me, I'm unstoppable.

So I give them the list and then—this is the hard part—if I feel myself slipping and wanting something, you got to make that call before you have it. I'm not always good at that. I've slipped up thousands of times, so I've learned to let myself off the hook. I don't condemn myself. I don't berate myself. I don't beat myself up, because for the most part, I'm batting in the high nineties, which is much better than most people.

Brian: That's fantastic, and you are touching on a lot of points that I often mention. Would you say that the accountability to your friends really helped push you to keep it up?

Mark: Absolutely! We check in with another comedian, Steve Mittleman, too; we check in and help each other every day. We say this is what our plan is and we do it for today. I can't tell you I'm not having pizza for the next thirty years, but I can tell you I'm not having it today.

Brian: That's a great attitude. One step at a time, right?

Mark: Yep, that's how I keep off the booze. That's how I keep off the cigars. That's how I keep off the dreck.

Brian: You mentioned as you were touring, how you would drink on the road and not remember being on tour for two weeks. My problem is when I tour, I eat. The unfortunate thing with eating is that you remember.

Your friend Jerry Seinfeld is well known for being thin. I know that he helped you get started in your weight loss. Was he there for you throughout the process?

Mark: Yeah. He did the foreword of my new book, but he's been on me to write up my little group as well.

You know, some people are naturally trim and they don't have to do anything, and we all hate those people. He exercises like a fiend. He exercises, like, six, seven days a week, with a massive amount of weights. He eats pretty good. He does some intermittent fasting. He knows the way I eat, and I think it's encouraged him a little to eat better, but he's got to work at it.

There's a little fat guy inside of me that's dying to come out all the time. He's alive and well, and he's waiting to go and order everything he can.

By the way, about the road: the road is difficult, but I've mastered it to a great degree with food. You don't have to drink and do drugs, but you do have to eat. For many years I did my own cooking on the road. I'd bring pots and a pan with me and a little stove and I would cook in the room. If there's a minibar, I call downstairs and make up a story. I need the alcohol out of the room and sometimes they don't want to do that. So if you tell them it's a religious thing, they have to do it. Then I stock my refrigerator with all kinds of food. I go to Whole Foods and I buy good, healthy foods. Sometimes I'll just eat canned food, I'll eat canned vegetables. I don't care about taste and satiating and all that crap. I just need to eat good, healthy stuff, and if that means sitting alone in a room and doing it, I'm fine with that.

Brian: Did your experience with alcohol help you with losing weight or controlling your diet?

Mark: There's no quitting. Like a good baseball player, a shortstop, you just try to cut off the first drink before it gets to the outfield and you start running around.

It's stronger than I am. Food's stronger, and it beat me, so one day at a time, I keep it at bay. That's all I can do. I can't pretend that I got it licked. Quitting the alcohol was the first thing for me, but a lot of people don't have that problem. So this is really the main crux of it. All these addictions are threefold diseases: physical, mental, and spiritual.

I was in therapy for seventeen years. It did nothing to keep me from drinking. I just had to wake up one day. That was it. I talked to a therapist for years about all kinds of shit and nothing.

There's an emptiness inside of me, and like for a lot of people who are addicted to things, it is insatiable and an endless pit that cannot be filled. I had to find something stronger than that to help me through. That's my connection to the spiritual. I meditate. I do transcendental meditation. Seinfeld got me involved with that too. He actually paid for my course. I exercise, and I'm a believer in God. So those three give me strength for one day.

In the Jewish Bible, when the Jews were going through the desert, God gave them manna from heaven for one day at a time. He didn't give them three weeks' worth; instead, every day he drops some food to them. So that's the way it is with me. I get enough power there to get through today. Tomorrow I'll deal with . . . I may not be alive tomorrow, who knows? So I don't have to worry about tomorrow.

Brian: My moment was the impending birth of my daughter. That was my wake-up call. I'm an older guy. I had my first kid at forty-five, and I was looking at life and thought that I might not make it to see her as a teenager. I doubt I'll see her go to college, but I'll be lucky to see her as a teenager.

How has losing the weight changed your life?

Mark: I used to be ashamed to go up on stage. I'm this fat guy. My shirt's hanging out, of course every time I tucked it in it would pop back out. I can't button my collar when I'm wearing a tie, it keeps popping open. I would sweat.

Now I go up, I'm trim. I got a couple of handmade, two-thousand-dollar suits. I look like a frigging billionaire, it's unbelievable. My hair is combed and I'm shaved. It gives me a real sense of well-being.

I was sick for many years, high blood pressure, high cholesterol; even at eighteen, I was diagnosed with high blood pressure.

That's pretty early on. I was always afraid I was going to drop dead at any given moment and have a stroke when I was fat. Now that I lost the weight, I don't really worry about it anymore. I've been relieved of the obsession with dying. That's a big deal.

I'm grateful for what I've done. I'm grateful for what I have. I was a late father too. I've got three boys. I was, like, forty years old when I had my first kid, and I couldn't play with them.

I didn't want to be one of those fathers to sit on the couch. "Kick the ball! Oh, I've got to get up? Forget it!" You know, just like you.

Brian: Has your comedy been influenced by losing the weight?

Mark: I never did fat jokes or any of that stuff. I just move better. I look better. When you hit the road, you better be in shape. As you get older, you're dragging your ass around airplanes and you can't lift the bag because your back hurts. The road is not a place for a guy out of shape.

I never want to gain it back. I know where it's going to end if I do, and it's not going to be pretty.

I'd rather be dead than force my family to have to take care of me. Something is going to happen one day. If I'm doing my best to take care of myself that's one thing, but if I stick them with this guy who didn't listen to a frigging thing his whole life, and now I'm in this chair and they've got to diaper me . . . When it's my fault, I'm going to feel a lot worse than if I did everything I could to take care of myself, and God forbid something happens. You know what I mean?

Brian: There's a difference between getting hit by a bus and getting hit by a buffet.

Mark: That's a great way to put it.

I was given this gift of a healthy body and I was lucky, because a lot of people aren't given that at birth. I want to return it in the best shape I can when it's time to give it back. I want to thank my higher-power guide and say, "Listen, I did the best I could with this temple you gave me."

Brian: Excellent. Mark, I want to thank you so much. Any closing comments you'd like to share with my readers?

Mark: One day at a time. There's really nothing you can't do, and I'm talking from experience. I've stopped so many horrific things just in this twenty-four-hour period. If you're struggling, you don't have to wait for tomorrow to make the change. You can start your day over right this minute. That's a concept that I learned. A lot of these people go, "I'll start tomorrow." No, start right this second. That's the only advice I can give.

Comedian Steve Mittleman Lost Fifty Pounds and Has Kept Most of Them Off for Thirty-Seven Years

I was still in high school when the movie *Roxanne*, starring Steve Martin, came out. It was a funny, heartwarming movie, and a memorable one. Around the same time, I started watching a lot of late-night TV, that is, whenever my parents let me, and I began to notice some of the supporting cast from *Roxanne* perform stand-up on shows like the *Tonight Show Starring Johnny Carson* or *An Evening at the Improv*. I didn't yet know Steve Mittleman by name, but there would be a moment of mild excitement when I'd see him come out on one of those stages. I'd yell to my brother, Jon, "That's the guy! That's the guy who said, 'I'm looking at a man who, when he washes his face, loses the bar of soap.'" His delivery of that line still makes me laugh.

Coincidentally, Steve Mittleman is also from Montreal. Not that I am, but I'm currently writing this in . . . ah, who cares—you get where I was going with that. Anyway, let's get to the interview.

Brian: At this point in the book, I'm reaching out to others to try to get some inspiration, so that's why I want to talk to some comedians who have lost weight.

Steve: I think comedians by nature are sort of philosophers a bit. I think they think things through a lot, so it's not a bad source in a way.

Brian: So how much weight have you lost?

Steve: I'd say between forty and fifty pounds. At my peak I didn't weigh myself, but I probably was somewhere between 220 to 230, and now I'm steadily around 180.

Brian: What prompted the weight loss?

Steve: Health and peace of mind, longevity, a better quality of life . . .

Brian: And how long have you been able to keep it off?

Steve: Well, that's been a bumpy road. I was in the mid-190s when COVID hit. We stopped eating out, and the fact that I wasn't eating sugar, oil, and salt from restaurants, it naturally came off because we don't have sugar, oil, and salt at home. Only a couple of times in the past thirty-seven years did I ever get up to the 220 mark again.

Brian: How did you drop the weight back then? I know it was a long time ago.

Steve: Mainly by upping the fruits and veggies, and reducing processed foods. Basically, it's common sense. You know, common sense never changes. I'm talking about for all of humanity. You are what you eat and you are what you don't eat. You said, how did I do that? It was upping the "best for me" stuff and lowering the "worst for me" stuff.

Brian: I like that you mentioned the common sense aspect, because one thing I mention early on is that everyone knows how to lose weight: You eat less and exercise more. That's something that we all know.

So how has your life improved by losing weight?

Steve: It's freedom. My dad had a stroke and four heart attacks; he died on his fourth heart attack. My mom had breast cancer, which turned to bone cancer, and died. The more I take care of myself, the less I have to worry about those foodborne diseases. Obesity is a foodborne disease.

And peace of mind. See that chair over there? I meditate in that chair. If you have weight on your stomach, you have a monkey on your back. Oh, I gotta write that down.

Brian: I'll be sure to put it in the book.

Steve: I like it. Quote me.

Brian: You had mentioned that you lost weight recently because of COVID limiting your opportunities to eat out. Something that I'd like to ask all the comics is, how do you maintain healthy habits when you're on the road?

Steve [imitating Rodney Dangerfield]: Hey, it ain't easy, Johnny.

I did exercise. Almost whatever town I was doing a comedy club in, or even a one-nighter, I would use the hotel gym. It helped me and grounded me, but I don't think it's really an element in weight loss. I think it's a gateway to "I love myself. I'm doing this loving thing. I'll make a loving choice when I'm eating."

If I could impart anything to you kids on the eating business, it is that food is 99 percent of the formula. You are what you eat.

We're not Olympic athletes. If this goes against your belief about what you do, I'm just sharing what I believe about what I do, but the truth is that food is 99 percent of it. Exercise is the unbelievable bonus icing on the cake.

Brian: Mm, cake.

Steve: What do I do on the road? I've probably eaten in fifty, sixty, seventy, or eighty Whole Foods and gotten salads. I generally try to eat healthier on the road. Unfortunately, when you do an event and there's a buffet, you gotta cherry-pick the best stuff there. It's not easy when unhealthy stuff's around.

It's so much easier when you're at home because you have an easy environment. If I am flying, I'll bring a giant thing of strawberries or a salad, stuff like that. When you're out of the house, it's best to seek out anything that replicates what's at home. That's the way to do it.

We live near Palm Springs and were recently in LA for three days. We ate out a few meals and did the best we could, but we did bring a lot of foods that we eat at home. My girlfriend and I eat the same, so we brought brown rice, cooked kale, and chopped salad.

Success leaves clues. These clichés, like "Common sense" and "Success leaves clues," are true. Replicate what worked before.

When I upped my veggies, upped my fruit, and upped my whole foods, and I cut back on crap, I got successful. So you live and learn from your time windows of success. And you go, "I'm gonna replicate what works."

When it comes to a diet or food plan, people always go, "I fell off the wagon." That's the lore of addiction. When you have a history of dopamine jolts from eating fatty or sugary or salty foods, your mind is going to yell, "I want to go back to that."

Comedian AC Valiante Has Lost Fifty Pounds Since the Start of the Pandemic

I met AC Valiante this summer in Montreal. He has been performing comedy for several years in Quebec, where he has his own weekly show, and will soon be entering a PhD program at McGill, making him yet another comedian with a doctorate. He was still working but had already managed to lose fifty pounds and keep them off for over a year.

Brian: How have you lost the weight?

AC: It is going to sound kind of cliché, but calories in and calories out. It's really about not eating too much. Ultimately it came down to that, respecting the laws of thermodynamics. I also do weight training—basic weights: biceps, triceps, back, shoulders, legs, bench press, stuff like that. I'm not much into cardio. It's not really my thing.

I've been struggling with my weight for quite a long time. I decided to make a change in my life right around the start of the pandemic. Being trapped at home for a while got me thinking about my life and my choices, and I decided that I needed to do something about it. I was at my heaviest around March 2020 when I was about 315 pounds.

Right around that time, my mom was diagnosed with cancer, so I started to take a real hard look at all the health decisions that I made. My mom had made some unhealthy choices in her life as well. She had been diabetic for a long time; she took medication that affected her kidneys and they shut down. And the medication that she was taking to counteract that may or may not have led to her developing cancer. I realized that I didn't want to follow the same path, so better late than never.

Brian: How has losing weight impacted your life?

AC: I started feeling better in my skin. I wasn't as tired waking up. I had a lot more energy. I started feeling better in my daily life. I started to fit better in my clothes, which was great. I always hated clothes shopping, and I always hated replacing my clothes because I had outgrown them. So going backward in my wardrobe actually felt pretty good. I'm now smaller than the clothes I was wearing five years ago, which is great. Let's just say it has also positively affected my relationship in a more . . . intimate manner. I may or may not be talking about banging.

Writer and Comedian Jonelle Larouche Lost Thirty Pounds by Giving Up Alcohol

Jonelle is originally from a small town in Northern Ontario, but I met her in Montreal. She is a freelance writer and aspiring comedian.

Brian: How have you lost your weight?

Jonelle: My weight loss journey started in January 2020. That's when I quit drinking. The weight came off immediately. I had been struggling to take it off for the past two years: running, busting my ass in the gym, and eating healthy during the week. But when the weekend came around, I'd drink wine from Friday to Sunday, ignoring the thousands of empty calories I was consuming. *There must be something wrong with this thing*, I thought every time I got off the scale, passive-aggressively kicking it back in its place.

Brian: What motivated the change?

Jonelle: I was on an emotional roller coaster. There were some unaddressed mental-health issues lurking beneath the surface. I was diagnosed with OCD and social anxiety. Every time we had plans to do something with people, I immediately felt the need to have drinks. You know, to calm my anxiety.

Brian: This is a social activity. Did you have a drink before this interview?

Jonelle: No, I haven't. I've been sober. I stopped drinking in January 2020, and I haven't [partaken] since.

Brian: How do you cope with anxiety without your go-to . . .?

Jonelle: My crutch? Exercise, meditation, reading funny books. Comedy would be another one. I think it's my new addiction. Writing. I need to be creating something to feel at peace. I've also started to wash my armpits multiple times before every social situation. Call it a new coping mechanism. I'm late for everything, but I guess it's better than getting drunk.

Brian: And that seems to work as well?

Jonelle: I've managed to keep the weight off, so I must be doing something right, but it's not easy. Some days I just wanna shove everything in my face. More specifically, a bottle of cabernet sauvignon with a side of carbs hiding under a heavy blanket of melted cheese. Losing weight is one thing; keeping it off is another challenge in itself.

Brian: How has your life improved by losing the weight?

Jonelle: I feel a lot more confident. With the weight gain came insecurities because I had never experienced being overweight. It was new to me and I didn't feel like myself.

When you start feeling better about yourself, it allows you to move forward and grow. I took some writing classes, which I never had the courage to do before. I also went to therapy and got to the bottom of my self-destructive thoughts and behaviors. I realized what I need to be happy. I'm more on the path to where I want to be as a person. I'm meeting people, like-minded people, like comedians. I fit in better with comedians and creatives. All crucial to staying fit, both mentally and physically.

Brian: What about writing? What kind of stuff do you like to write about?

Jonelle: Right now I'm focused on my personal journey from childhood on. The screenplay I'm working on is a dramedy about the evolution of a human being throughout a lifetime. It's never too late to make changes. My mother went back to school when she was forty-five to be an addictions counselor. Witnessing this was very inspiring for me. I want to help people with things I've been through, my experiences, all the work I've done through therapy, reading books on psychology, and my vast collection of inspirational quotes.

Comedian Trevin Verduzco Has Lost Eighty-Five Pounds with the Help of a Weight Loss Clinic

I don't remember officially meeting Trevin Verduzco in Colorado. I was in Durango working on my last book in and started seeing him around at open mics. There was no handshake, no formal introduction; we became acquainted through osmosis. Comedy scenes are like that: as you watch each other perform over time you come to know people. I never thought he was physically huge, but he was heavy enough to be noticeable. Two years later I returned to Durango and his weight loss was dramatic. He looked great and seemed much happier as well.

Brian: When you started doing comedy, were you overweight?

Trevin: I was. I have been overweight for most of my life. When I was in college, I got on a little bit of a weight loss spree and I managed to get it under control. But as I've gotten older, typically as men enter into their early twenties, issues with mental health tend to manifest, and for me that was depression. Combine that with a pretty brutal schedule and trying to study computer science. It resulted in a very negative feedback loop where I'd feel like shit, so I'd eat like shit to make myself feel better, and then I'd feel more like shit because . . . yeah. Then I'd eat even more.

Brian: How have you lost the weight?

Trevin: I got started with the local weight loss clinic, and they really helped me pick up on a lot of different things and reevaluate my relationship with food. There were three key things that I would say really helped me drop my weight. The first was changing my diet. I eliminated carbs and I eliminated high-sugar foods, including certain vegetables. The second thing was food journaling, being able to keep track of what I was eating, how much and when, and have a log of that that I would not type digitally but handwrite. By handwriting what I'd eaten, it really helped it sink in and helped me keep track of everything. Third was increasing my activity. At the time, I was in a very bad bout of depression. I was unemployed for a month and a half. Basically, I got right back on the horse, started getting more into waiting tables. I hit a point where I was working three jobs. I would be on my feet for at least thirty hours a week, walking around and lifting heavy boxes, things like that.

Brian: You mentioned cutting out certain vegetables. What vegetable didn't make the diet?

Trevin: The thing is, certain vegetables are very dense in sugar. Bell pepper was one of them, as in sweet bell peppers. Carrots are a huge one. Carrots are delicious. I love carrots to death, but carrots are basically candy. They have a ton of sugar in them. And they are terrible for you when you're in that phase of weight loss.

Brian: How has losing all that weight changed your life?

Trevin: I don't think a lot of people focus on how diet really impacts the hormonal balance of the person and how that can impact your mental health and your ability to manage stress. When I was at my biggest, I was eating a lot of high-carb foods, a lot of high-sugar foods. I was an emotional wreck. The slightest thing could happen and it would send me into a fucking spiral. I would freak out. I was not able to manage stress well, but once I got past that and got a month or two into my weight loss journey, I noticed that those things didn't affect me as much. I was able to keep a much cooler head on my shoulders. I was able to navigate the daily hardships of life a lot more effectively. I was able to plan and strategize better. That's one of the more low-key things that I don't see mentioned much when it comes to weight loss. Of course, there's more obvious stuff: boosting confidence that comes from getting more attention, being able to wear clothes that you've always wanted to wear, and things like that. But those are more outward-facing things that help improve and change your life, whereas the more interesting stuff, the stuff that I pulled more from, was more inward facing.

The big thing is being able to manage stress better and being able to develop new coping mechanisms that are a lot healthier for dealing with that stress instead of going to my old default of comfort eating.

Brian: That's awesome. What sort of coping mechanisms do you utilize now?

Trevin: The key thing was trying to find ways to practice mindfulness in the brief moments that you have throughout your daily life. Because like you, I'm a very busy guy. I mean, four jobs a week. They're all part-time jobs, but that doesn't leave you with a lot of free time to get really into painting or to build models or stuff like that. Just being able to identify small things I can do throughout my day to help myself destress, like taking a moment in between my shifts to go enjoy a nice black coffee and sit down, read a little bit of a book, practice writing in my comedy notebook, or even small things like instead of going for the candy bar when I'm having a rough night at tables, heading out back and punching a trash can while screaming "Fuck!" at the top of my lungs. Stuff like that.

Brian: I would never have guessed that a punching a trash can would be as satisfying as eating a candy bar.

Trevin: Oh, trust me. It is way more satisfying.

Comedian Mark Evans Lost One Hundred Pounds Thanks to Intermittent Fasting

I first met Mark at a comedy club in Cocoa Beach, Florida. I was a few years into my speaking career and had a seminar at a nearby hotel when I popped in and asked the club manager if I could get a guest spot that night. He told me to ask the headliner, which was Mark, so I went over and introduced myself. Mark was nice enough to give me a spot in the show that night, one that led to my getting booked there as a feature the next year and as a headliner after that. Mark had been a working comedian for about twenty years at that point. I was probably a decent opener for him, as we were both big guys and I got to test the durability of the stage before he went on.

Although our tour schedules don't have us crossing paths very often, we have kept in touch over the years, and thanks to social media I have seen him and his wife undergo a dramatic weight loss.

Brian: Can you tell me a bit about your history with being overweight?

Mark: I grew up an athlete. I think what really first got me was when I got to be twenty-one, I was still playing semi-pro soccer, but I was old enough to drink beer. So, uh, that. I never really overate; I just didn't eat right. When I was playing soccer, I could eat at McDonald's and it meant nothing, 'cause it would fall off me. But as I played ball less, and with getting older, I kept my same eating habits. I wasn't a fall-down drunk, but beer didn't help. And the weight slowly crept on. Then ten, fifteen, or twenty years later, it's like, where did this come from, you know? It wasn't an overnight problem. I grew up skinny, but it was when I quit being as active and didn't adjust my eating habits. That was the mistake.

Brian: How do you manage eating on the road? Do you think touring contributed to your weight accumulation?

Mark: Oh definitely, because it's really hard to eat right. It's almost impossible not to eat fast food, because when you're traveling six, seven, eight hours a day between gigs, you don't really have time to try to seek out a place that is very healthy.

Brian: How have you lost the weight?

Mark: My wife started intermittent fasting first, and two weeks later I joined her because, well, I didn't have any choice. Do you remember what Samuel Jackson said in *Pulp Fiction*? He goes, "My girlfriend's a vegetarian, which pretty much means that I'm a vegetarian too now." Same thing. And it was the easiest thing I ever did. I would only eat in a four-hour window, usually from 4 p.m. to 8 p.m. The beauty of intermittent fasting was that I could eat whatever I wanted to, and it worked. One of the things you could do outside of that four-hour window was drink black coffee, water, or unsweetened tea. When I was on the road, I could stop and get the dollar McDonald's unsweetened tea and not eat anything until the four o'clock window opened up.

It was easy for me because it didn't take that long to adjust. I rarely eat more than one meal a day anyway. So that part wasn't hard to adjust to. And when you knew you could eat whatever you wanted and the weight was falling off you, I didn't mind at one o'clock going, "OK, my window's gonna open at four, but I wanna get a pizza." So I could have a goal and it was worth waiting for. If it was wait three hours and then I got to eat a keto meal or something, there's no incentive.

Brian: How long did it take you to drop a hundred pounds?

Mark: Nine months. It went fast. Intermittent fasting, I can't speak enough for it. A lot of people think it's a starvation diet, but I don't see it that way. They call it breakfast in the morning because you're breaking your fast of the night. I just take longer fasts. And of course, when you have more to lose, you lose it quicker. When you get down to the nitty-gritty, that takes a little more time. But that's with any diet.

Brian: That's a nice thing about being huge: you cut out one meal and you're gonna lose weight.

Mark: Like I say, I could have flossed and lost five pounds at one point.

Brian: And what about the beer drinking?

Mark: I say I drink, but I hardly ever drink anymore. At gigs, the only time I'll even think about having a drink is if it's one of the gigs where the club is inside the hotel and all I gotta do is walk to my room, I might have a drink afterward. But then at my age I get to the point where I like waking up feeling good tomorrow morning. The younger comics would want me to go out and party. I go, "No, somebody's gotta be able to get you outa jail." But you know, we're down here in Florida now, and it's fun to sit at the pool and have a couple beers. And the beauty of it is, two or three beers and I've got a strong buzz.

Brian: I stopped too. I'm not telling people that I don't drink, but the reality is I don't drink.

Mark: That's pretty much where I am now.

Comedian Kieran Atkins Lost Forty-Five Pounds by Overcoming Impulsive Behavior

I have been running a comedy writing group on Facebook for years. It began with a small group of San Francisco comedians who would meet on a regular basis and give each other feedback on jokes we were working on. When I moved away and started touring, it became a virtual tool and has since grown to be one of the largest comedy-related groups on Mark Zuckerberg's hard drive. At one point I felt as if it had gotten a little too big to be all that helpful to any individual writer, as there were more posts than feedback. It was in this context that a handful of London comedians, including Kieran Atkins, joined as part of a plot to imperialize American comedy. Stand-up comedy is an American art form, but it is not uniquely American. There are some widely known differences between British and American humor, and neither is better than the other. The Brits trolled my group, posting intentionally awful puns while asking for feedback, which pissed off many of the more serious members, and I loved them for it. By shaking it up, they created activity and prompted many of the better writers to come out of the shadows. At least for a little while.

In the summer before the pandemic, I took Sarah and Alyssa to Europe for a month. Our trip started and ended in London, and that same gang of comedians booked a comedy show for me at a pub in the South Bank. I got to meet Kieran, Julius, and the others in person, and we had an awesome show followed by a fun night at the bar before taking the tube back to our hotel in our "stabby" neighborhood.

Unfortunately, being overweight is also an American characteristic, but it is not uniquely American. Before I arrived, I knew that a couple of these blokes were overweight, thanks again to the code that made Zuckerberg a billionaire, but standing side by side with these guys, I came to realize that there is a big difference between American fat and English fat. Thankfully, in the time since, both Kieran and I have been slimming down for our countries.

Brian: Tell me a bit about your history as somebody who has struggled with weight loss.

Kieran: I'm thirty-eight years old, and I began gaining weight when I was around nine or ten. Of course, in England back in the late 1980s and early 1990s, there weren't really that many fat people around at all.

In my early to mid-teens—because at that age you want to meet girls and that kind of thing, you have to have a ripped six-pack, you gotta be six foot two, and you gotta have a massive dick—I realized that I could do most of those things apart from having a ripped six-pack and being six foot two. When I began thinking about this problem, I thought the way to lose weight was to exercise a hell of a lot and starve. There's always been this diction, if you will: "Move more, eat less." Well, if I ate less and I lost weight, that would last for about a week, and then I'd go back to eating normal again. That lasted for about twenty years. What is interesting is I didn't pick up on it. I thought, *Well, that's just me and my genes and that's the way it is.* Interestingly, during that time I became quite successful in a particular sport in which being able to gain weight wasn't a bad thing. That was being a powerlifter.

Brian: When you said you were in a sport that wasn't affected by being overweight, I thought maybe you were talking about sumo wrestling or something.

Kieran: I'm told that eating is now a sport in the US.

Brian: Yeah, eating competitions are a thing here. It's ridiculous, and ironically fat guys aren't winning them. So what prompted you to decide to lose weight?

Kieran: Over time, you realize there are issues. You're perhaps ignored by the female sex for being overweight, or you're seen as the funny guy of the group. It's interesting, because one has to be that funny guy in order to be seen.

Brian: I feel bad for fat guys who aren't funny.

Kieran: I've been trying for twenty-plus years and I'm still on that journey. I realized that at times I may not necessarily be in control of how I eat. I didn't have an addiction, it wasn't that, and I didn't binge eat. It was impulsive eating. This occurred to me during the lockdown. I began to research ADHD and discovered that I tick all of the boxes. I realized this is how my impulsive traits manifest, through eating. As a comedian, ADHD has proven very helpful to say the least, especially at times when you're thinking on the fly, when you have to think very, very quickly. Sometimes you can do a forty-five-minute show but only have about ten minutes' worth of material.

I discovered that impulsive eating led to more impulsive eating. I began to strictly log everything I ate, and I avoided foods that I knew gave me a high reward feeling. Certain types of carbs or cheeses, that kind of thing.

Brian: It's interesting that you mentioned ADHD. That's exactly how I got overweight as well. Poor impulse control and forgetting that I've already eaten. How much weight have you lost?

Kieran: I've lost in total now forty-five pounds, and I have another forty to lose. This is a very tricky situation, because my whole identity, my self-perception, has been built around me being fat. This is very unnerving, but there's a part of me, I think this unconscious part of me, that doesn't want to let that go. Because that has been the identity for a long time.

Brian: Me too. I hit a hundred pounds and then I've been going up and down, fluctuating around the same ten pounds. It's been difficult. My brain thinks of me as a fat person, not a potential skinny person.

Kieran: I've been trying to lose weight for twenty-plus years, and each time I did was probably duc to an event—a breakup, not getting the job interview that I wanted, or wanting to look good for a holiday. When you think about it, most of these drives revolve around shame as a motivator, which is not a compassionate motivation to lose weight. I'm going to show them by doing this! Right. It ends up not working.

Brian: The negative emotion that's motivating you doesn't last very long. You start to get over it and whatever, there's other jobs, there's other girls out there. It doesn't stick. So how did you lose the forty-five pounds?

Kieran: By now having a very firm cognitive understanding of my behavior. I realized what I was doing. I had this metacognition in place where if I had a certain urge or impulse, I needed to create a space where I could decide what to do. There is an element of mindfulness to it. Meditation gave me a full amount of cognitive space to make that micro decision. Do I go to the fridge or not? When I'm in the supermarket, do I buy the chicken breasts or do I buy the chocolate bars? It's a no-brainer. So there was that cognitive space, and mindfulness meditation helped me considerably. Also understanding of my behavior, as once I knew the patterns, I was able to work with it. I also realized that it is OK to go off the rails once every now and then as long as you pick yourself back up off the floor and be gentle with yourself. So that's been my experience of it so far.

Brian: How has losing weight affected your life?

Kieran: Very positively! I seem to be more successful in the workplace. I have a lot more mental energy to get things done despite the ADHD, which is something that I will address later. In terms of my love life, I'm doing way better now. In terms of my sport, powerlifting, I'm actually becoming stronger, because there is a recompositioning effect: I'm able to lose fat and replace it with muscle mass. Probably in two years, I'll be competing again at quite a serious level due to that. So that's really good.

Brian: How much can you lift?

Kieran: Bench-press is 140 kilos [308 pounds], I'm squatting 220 kilos [485 pounds], and deadlift 250 [551 pounds]. Ideally, I would like to be able to squat three times my weight. That is the gold standard.

Comedian Jennifer Anderson Lost Eighty Pounds by Kickboxing!

Prior to writing this book I had never met Jennifer Anderson in person. Comedians tend to be heavily into social networking, and at some point she and I connected, probably each of us thinking the other was a fan. Over the years, I did become a fan of hers online, as I really enjoy her humor. When I learned that she had lost a lot of weight and shared her story on national TV, I knew that I had to reach out to her for this book.

Brian: Can you tell me a bit about your weight loss?

Jennifer: Well, which time? I probably lost a hundred pounds the first time, and gained, like, eighty of that back from severe depression. Then I lost maybe fifty since college, gained that back, and then went on the TV show and lost eighty pounds.

Brian: What was the TV show?

Jennifer: *This Time Next Year*. It was to inspire people to be able to do anything on their own in a year. Say you began it on September 12, you would have to have reached your goal by the next September 12.

Brian: How have you lost the weight?

Jennifer: So after crying myself to sleep several nights, staring at myself in the mirror and wishing I could change my body, I kickboxed every single day. Then I did Zumba for probably two hours in the morning. Then I changed everything to a Paleo diet. I don't think I got the last twenty pounds off, because at eighty pounds lost they wanted me to go skydiving and I was like, no. No, this giant bird is not gonna skydive. You're not going to push me out of a plane. I'm not going to Sesame Street. No, thank you.

Brian: Did you start kickboxing for the show?

Jennifer: I've been kickboxing since I was twenty-five. When I did the show, I was thirty-six. So I went back to the thing that I loved, which was kickboxing. And then I discovered Zumba, because it's so high in cardio. I loved that so much. I started teaching it too.

Brian: So kickboxing wasn't a new activity.

Jennifer: No, I've been beating the crap outa people for years. It was just kinda my thing.

Brian: That's a different book. How about your diet?

Jennifer: It was a Paleo diet where you cut out carbs and kind of eat natural. You eat more whole grains, veggies, and clean meat. So no In-N-Out Burger or anything like that. Taco Bell? No. Anything tasty? No, go outside and eat a tree.

Brian: I don't know if I could live like that.

Jennifer: Why did they take away the Mexican pizza?

Brian: It's funny you mention Taco Bell. There's a part of my book where I go on extensively about it.

Jennifer: It's the best junk food ever.

Brian: How did losing the weight affect your life?

Jennifer: I ditched diabetes. I was prediabetic, so I got that under control. I got my cholesterol under control. I was able to go back to theme parks and fly on a plane. I hadn't flown in five or six years. They flew me to Las Vegas, where they wanted me to jump out of the plane to Vegas. But I was like, we're not insured for that, so no. But I got to go on a plane to Las Vegas. My first plane in five years. It was a huge confidence booster too, which was awesome.

Brian: How else has losing weight affected your life?

Jennifer: I was able to perform again. I didn't like performing big because I do so much physical stuff. So I was able to go back to stand-up comedy. I was confident in making my jokes, and I felt really good onstage. Going up there as a giant person, you feel like

Chris Farley, and I didn't want to go that way.

Brian: I didn't realize your weight got in the way of your stand-up. You didn't do any fat jokes?

Jennifer: I always did tall jokes, because I thought that was more important than fat jokes.

Brian: Do you get recognized on the street from your TV appearances?

Jennifer: Every now and then. I got recognized at a Subway of all places, and they're like, "Oh my God, aren't you Jennifer Anderson?" Yes, yes I am.

Brian: Do you feel obligated to order something healthy in that situation?

Jennifer: Yeah. I'm like, I'll take the veggie stuff. No, I don't want the meatball with extra cheese. You can take that away. I totally want wheat bread with extra cucumber. I'll take that. Thank you, random stranger.

Brian: So weight loss got you back onstage, gave you confidence, and you feel healthier. Are you still kickboxing?

Jennifer: Oh yeah. I still have to get my rage out.

Comedian Erik Escobar Lost Over One Hundred Pounds Because He Had a Toothache

In 2014 I was still living in West Hollywood but spending a lot of my time on the road. Through word of mouth, I learned that a comedian was organizing the first comedy festival in Boise, Idaho. I applied and was fortunate enough to be accepted. The festival was amazing, particularly given it was its first year, and is still one of my favorite festival memories. When it came time to submit for the second year, I gladly threw my hat in the ring. I was lucky to be selected again, and soon after the roster was announced, I was contacted by a young comedian named Erik Escobar. We had never previously met, but we both lived in the Los Angeles area and were planning to drive to Idaho. We decided to travel together to share expenses and use our various connections along the route to make a mini-tour out of the trip. We booked gigs in Reno on the way up and in Sacramento on the way down, and throughout it all we became pretty good friends despite the twenty-year age difference. Since then, we've bumped into each other on the road a few times.

Brian: Tell me a bit about your history as an overweight person.

Erik: In high school I was a big kid. I wasn't super, super big, but I was pretty big. I think a lot of it was because I was a bit of a latchkey kid. I would snack when I got home from school, like crazy. Snacking became a coping mechanism for me. Not that I had any severe trauma or anything, but it made me feel good if I was bored.

Both of my parents worked, and when they came home from work every day, they didn't want to cook. So we would eat out a lot. We had a lot of fast food growing up. I think that because we ate out so much, every opportunity to eat was kind of like a celebration. It was like, why are you getting a salad? Get a burger! Get a bacon cheeseburger! Get whatever you want! Because of that, I really gained this mentality that whatever I do, I want to make sure I get the most out of it. When I was eating, I wanted to get the biggest meal. I wanted to get the coolest thing, the biggest thing.

And that's something that stuck with me for a very long time. I would go out on the road and it would be like I don't know when I'll be in Denver again, I don't know when I'll be in Idaho again, in San Francisco, so let's eat everything in this town. Eating became this weird mentality. I gotta eat as much as I can because if I don't I might not have it again. I need to take advantage of the situation.

Brian: How big did you get at your highest point, and how much did you lose?

Erik: Whether I was gaining or losing weight, I was never one to really weigh myself that often. I didn't have a scale. But I definitely feel my biggest was probably just over 300, probably hovering around 310 or 315. Right now, I'm between 180 and 185. I kind of hover in that range.

Brian: That's amazing and definitely an achievement. What prompted the weight loss?

Erik: I think it was December 2019. I had a toothache. If anyone has ever had tooth problems, it sucks. I would rather have a broken back or a broken nose than tooth pain, because it stays with you all day. You can't really get over it. It sucks. I finally went to a dentist.

I was like, "Something's up with my molar. It's constantly in pain. I can't think. I can't focus. I can't sleep." And they're like, "We can repair it, but we need to get your vitals." And my blood pressure was recognized as super high. So they're like, "We can't do anything unless you get your blood pressure in order." And I was like, "This *sucks*."

I'm a comedian. I didn't have health insurance. I hadn't seen a doctor in three years. How do I even fix this? I ended up going to this free clinic and they gave me some blood pressure medication. I was like, "How long do I take this before I'm good?" And they're like, "Oh, this you don't stop. Like every day you have to take a pill for the rest of your life if you want your blood pressure in order. If you stop taking it, you could die."

I think when that moment happened, it was a big kick in the butt.

Brian: How have you lost the weight?

Erik: I was doing more of a low-carb diet, drinking a lot more water, exercising a little more, but I really feel the pandemic jumpstarted the weight loss. I got off the road, I was at home, and

I stopped eating after eight, nine o'clock, whereas before I would always eat at ten o'clock.

I feel like getting off the road forced me to not eat late at night, forced me to make my own meals, and by being in one location I was able to drink more water, which is a big deal. When I look at my last thirty years of life, I didn't drink water for shit. Like I didn't even know that was an option! Now I try to drink roughly a gallon a day.

Brian: Now that you are back on the road, how are you managing?

Erik: When you are pushing 310 pounds and you wake up every day, you might feel a little "Whatever," but that is how it is. Now that I've lost the weight, I wake up feeling more energized and not as sluggish, not as hungover. If I eat horribly for a night and I drink, like, ten beers and have a bacon cheeseburger and a slice of pizza, I'll wake up the next morning and I feel it for the next two or three days. If I'm being good and I have maybe one beer and a salad for dinner, I wake up in the morning feeling good and refreshed. And that's a big motivator.

You're not at home. You're sleeping on couches or you're sleeping in friends' basements. You're doing twelve-hour drives. All this crazy stuff just to get to gigs and work it. So anything that I can do to just feel not shitty and feel not worse on top of that, it's great.

Maintaining a low-carb diet on the road isn't that hard. It really is a forced lifestyle change you have to make. I can't look at every meal on the road and be like, I don't know when I'm going to be in New England again, so I better get fourteen lobster rolls.

I love eating and I love food, but I'm OK eating just the lobster or going to breakfast and having bacon and eggs, no toast. Whenever I go to McDonald's I'll get a sausage muffin with no muffin. And it's great: egg, cheese, and sausage. It's wonderful.

After a couple of weeks, you don't even think about it. You just kind of get into it. It is difficult. It'll be very difficult for the first few weeks or so. But after that it is going to get easier every day.

Brian: How has losing the weight affected your life?

Erik: You know what? There are parts of it I kind of hate, I really do. I was a single guy for many years, and when I was pushing three hundred, I feel like I didn't have game. You know what I mean? You approach a girl in the bar and they're like, you're a creeper. Over the past year, I have been seeing this amazing, beautiful, wonderful partner. We just got engaged. I love her so much. But for the four- or five-month period when I was single and skinny, it was great. Women would talk to me, they would approach me. I would get hit up after shows by women. Girls would ask me out and I was like, I'm the same person. I'm the same weird, goofy person. Being a big guy, there was this social stigma, and when you lose weight out of nowhere, they're like, "Hey, what's up?" It's so weird to experience that, and I kind of hate it because everyone's a beautiful person. You know what I mean?

Comedian Dave DeLuca Lost 110 Pounds by Walking Throughout New York City

I have known comedian Dave DeLuca for almost fifteen years. In fact, as of this writing, he is the only person other than Sarah and my brother, Jon, to be mentioned by name in all three of my books, a fact that I can only assume he is now including on his résumé.[110] Not even Alyssa can make that claim, although to be fair she didn't exist when I was writing the first book.

Dave and I met in San Francisco early in my comedy career. I had been running shows at my club for a while when he came in and introduced himself as having just arrived back in California from New York. He was funny, but more importantly he was nice, and we got along well, so we worked together a lot for the next couple of years up until the closing of my comedy club. When we both decided to move to Los Angeles at the same time, he became my first roommate since college.

We lived together for a few years, until a beautiful redhead convinced me to start a life with her (redheads can be very persuasive like that), and got along really well. We shared the same love of food, but Dave was a relentless exerciser. He balanced his calories with a lot of physical activity, something I tried unsuccessfully

110 Because of course Sarah and Jon do.

to join him in. He was always in good shape; he even booked an appearance on the TV show *Brooklyn Nine-Nine* because he was the same size costume as a cast member who got sick one week. I guess that is why I didn't immediately think to interview him for this book.

Brian: We've known each other a long time, and I've always known you to be thin and athletic, but onstage . . .

Dave: I'm beautiful.

Brian: I wouldn't go that far.

Dave: I saw you looking when we lived together. . . . [He says this while grinning and winking at me.]

Brian: Onstage you had always talked about losing weight and being fat. Can you tell me a bit about your history of being overweight?

Dave: I was a really athletic kid. I did a lot of sports and I ate like a dump truck. I was a competitive swimmer, I played competitive tennis, and, until about the age of eighteen, I could literally devour, if not one, possibly two large pizzas all to myself and not gain an ounce. I was thin and wiry for a long time.

When I was fifteen, I started going to the emergency room because something was going on in my leg. It took about three or four years to figure out I had a benign tumor underneath my left quad. When I was going into my senior year in college, they finally did the surgery to pull the whole thing out, and I spent the next two months with my leg straight out in a splint. I couldn't bend it. I couldn't do anything. Then I spent another year doing rehab and physical therapy, trying to get my strength back. I wasn't playing tennis, I stopped playing soccer, nothing. I had turned twenty-one, so I was able to drink, *and* I was also going through a bad breakup with somebody who I'd thought I was going to be with for the rest of my life. I was depressed about the whole situation, but in retrospect, I'm glad it didn't work out. Gotta take a shot at the ex when you can, right? [He's laughing to himself now.]

Anyway, I wasn't going to a lot of classes and if I did I would stop on the way home, pick up a pizza, get junk food like McDonald's or Taco Bell, and then sit and watch cable. I would just sit there and do nothing but drink and eat, and it wasn't healthy. And that continued after college. Perhaps because I knew I couldn't play competitively anymore, I wasn't even trying to play tennis or other sports, or really do anything.

Brian: From your peak, about how much weight did you lose?

Dave: I was 292 at my peak. After deciding to lose the weight I got down to 182, which was the lightest I've been since before college. I feel I'm a little heavy now, floating between 210 and 215, but I'm actually at a good weight for my age. I'm almost forty-five. And, I know, I look fantastic! I showered just for you, even though this is for a book and over video chat. Anyway, I'm at kind of an ideal weight for somebody my age, but I still want to get a little slimmer and toned. But it's been tough this last year with COVID and everything.

Brian: I know a lot of us gained a little during the past couple of years, but overall how long have you been managing your weight?

Dave: Fifteen years.

Brian: How did you lose that weight?

Dave: Calorie counting. I started slow. I changed my diet. I didn't drink for a year. I didn't buy sweets—well, I did, but if I bought something like that, like ice cream, I would have, like, two pints of ice cream and that would be my calories for the day.

Brian: I've had those days. I count calories too, and a bowl of ice cream is like, well, that's all I'm eating today.

Dave: Exactly! I was very strict. I had all my meals planned out. I incorporated a lot of vegetables. I would do vegetables and chili for just about every meal, and work in a protein bar for a midday snack. I kept myself at under fifteen hundred calories a day, which isn't healthy, but it's effective.

Then I started walking. I lived in New York City, and there was a lot of walking involved getting to and from work and going to lunch. On top of walking to and from work, I would walk for an hour after work while I listened to an audiobook. Then slowly I started doing other exercises, and I started playing tennis again. And that was something I could do all day and not be hungry at all because I was having fun. I could play for six hours a day on the weekend, easy.

I took up running when we moved to Los Angeles. Now I run about five miles a day. Sometimes I do seven to nine. And I hate running! I never wanted to be a runner, and I don't consider myself a runner now, but I do it. Not because I enjoy it, but because I want to get laid.

Brian: One of my favorite jokes of yours is very simple. It's about why you wanted to lose weight.

Dave: Yeah. It's part of a bigger bit, but the part I think you're hinting at is: "I used to be a hundred pounds heavier than I am right now. Then one day I decided I don't like to sweat when I make a sandwich!"

Brian: That's hilarious. That must have been a really big sandwich.

Dave: Giant sandwich! Have you tried spreading a foot long of mayo? It's not easy!

Brian: When you lost the weight, how did that impact your life?

Dave: It makes an enormous difference. I have a bunch of material about losing the weight. Another one of my jokes is, "The reason I lost the weight is to get laid, because I'm not rich and nobody wants to fuck the poor, fat guy." But it's true. And I think the biggest thing is that it does a lot for your self-confidence.

I'm forty-five and I still look pretty good! [He grins, winks at me again, and chuckles.] Anyway, when I lost the weight, it was immediate. When I got back from New York I was at a bar in the Bay Area where I knew the bouncer. I handed him my ID with a photo of me as fat, and he looked at it and wouldn't let me in. He was like, "I know this guy; this isn't you. What are you trying to pull? Are you his younger brother or something?"

I played it off. Instead of saying, "Dude it's me," I said that's my ID. It was a couple of minutes before he realized it was, and he was blown away. People were telling me that I looked younger, and I felt it. I realized that I felt and looked older when I was heavy. And the more I lost, the younger I felt.

My sex life also got better and at the same time I was able to enjoy sex more. And it's not just that I was able to have more of it, but I also wasn't exhausted during it. I still sweat, but now it's more because I'm doing acrobatic shit! Instead of trying to take off the shirt and going, "Oh God! Hold on! I gotta take a break. I just, I can't get it over my head right now!" I think I'm gonna have to use that onstage!

But yeah, it's improved my day-to-day life! Like going up stairs was a hassle when you're heavy. I have less hindrances now and I'm able to enjoy the things I want to do. If I'm exhausted at the end of the day it's because I did a ton, not because I sat on the couch and ate too much.

Brian: When we lived together, it seemed like the majority of your day was spent out on our porch jumping rope. Was that something you started early on?

Dave: I started doing it in New York. Jumping rope was a tennis thing. It's for footwork, and tennis is why I originally did it when I was younger. When I stopped playing tennis, obviously I didn't keep jumping rope, but it's good cardio. It gets the whole body involved, and for me it's a little lower impact on my knees. I actually haven't been jumping rope for a while now. About six months ago, they started construction at my place, so in lieu of jumping rope, I swim. I do anywhere from 100 to 150 laps—which is about two to three miles—at a time. But I want to go back to jumping rope because it's something that you can put on headphones and do. It's not the best for weight loss, but it's really good for fitness.

Brian: I remember one time jumping rope outside our West Hollywood apartment gave you a boost to your self-esteem.

Dave: Yeah! One that you overheard yourself! One day when I was jumping, and keep in mind when you're walking by on the street you can look into the garage and see somebody jumping rope for hours on end. Seriously! Someone could walk past, go down to the store, come back, and I could still be there. Anyway, there was this really nice guy who I had seen plenty of times before, walking his dog, and he'd look in and see me jumping, like, "What's going on over there?" One day, I'm finishing up, and as I'm walking to go back into our apartment, he comes up to me and says, "I just have to tell you you're the most gorgeous, good-looking man on the planet," and then scurried off, just ran away. I think he got embarrassed or something.

So I came into the apartment and I walked upstairs and was going to shower and change, and you're standing there. And I'm like, "You're not gonna believe what just happened!" And you looked at me and said, "You're the most gorgeous, good-looking man on the planet!" And we laughed about it. But honestly, it was incredibly flattering and told me that my work was paying off. That really made my day for a while. I felt great about myself. There's really no downside to it whatsoever.

Comedian ANT Lost Almost Seventy Pounds After Trying Nearly Everything

Dave DeLuca and I lived in West Hollywood at almost the perfect location for a couple of comedians. We were on a street perpendicular to Sunset and halfway between the Sunset Strip and Santa Monica Boulevard. This put us an easy walk from the major comedy clubs like the Laugh Factory, the Hollywood Improv, and the Comedy Store, with many second-tier clubs and comedy rooms also in close proximity. However, with so many venues to perform stand-up comedy in greater Los Angeles, there was, and will always be, way more comedians wanting stage time. Which is why Dave and I would often drive all over Southern California looking for places to practice our craft despite living in such a prime location.

By far the closest club to us was the Comedy Store, a legendary club that I loved as a comedy fan, revered after I became a comedian, and hardly worked when I finally moved to LA. That isn't to say that I didn't enjoy my performances there. I loved and appreciated every single time I was able to get on any of those stages (there are three), but as a comic without any major TV or movie appearances, it would be a while before I would become one of their regular performers. I didn't want to drive out of town every night, so it was clear that I needed to find another option.

One night, after leaving The Store,[111] I walked across the street to the since closed (and demolished) House of Blues. There was a band playing that I was interested in checking out, Detroit Diesel Power, and they were amazing. They had a traditional rock sound but were uniquely fronted by a female singer, Regina Zernay, who also played the most hardcore upright bass I have ever seen. Anyway, after having my face melted for a solid hour or so, I looked around and thought to myself, *I wonder if this place would ever host a comedy show?*

The next day I followed up with the manager, and soon Dave DeLuca and I were hosting a weekly comedy showcase at the House of Blues. Between the two of us, we were able to book a wide variety of comedians and of course give ourselves a regular opportunity to perform within walking distance of our apartment. One of the performers Dave booked was a comedian he met in New York who goes by the name ANT. Prior to working with him, I had seen him on *Last Comic Standing* and maybe a few late-night talk shows, so I was thankful he graced our stage and killed it. He was in good shape, and I knew that he had also hosted a show called *Celebrity Fit Club* on VH-1, so when someone recommended I talk to him for this book, I was a little surprised.

Brian: When we last worked together, I don't remember you having excess body weight. Can you tell me a bit about that?

ANT: Like a lot of people with mental health problems, I have struggled with weight my whole life. Meaning, I didn't know the underlying issues behind why I ate like I did. I didn't know I

111 Cool kids just call it "The Store."

was fat until my niece, when she was ten years old, said, "Uncle ANT, you look like a tomato wearing a belt!" Ouch! Kids don't lie. And that was the first time I ever took a hard look at my weight.

You're going to hear from lots of comedians. They lost weight with diet and exercise. Yeah, yeah, yeah . . . not me. I'm always looking for the easier, softer way. Surgery was always the easier, softer way. So I've had liposuction seven times.

Brian: Wow!

ANT: Well, first I did the Zone diet through a food delivery service. The food came, it was very, very bland. So I called the company up and they said, "Oh, well spice it up for taste." So I started spicing it up with pizza, burritos, and chalupas, and then wondered why I wasn't losing weight.

Then I discovered liposuction. Now, most people use liposuction to sculpt the body. I used it to drop weight. I went to a doctor in LA who does a lot of famous people, and he asked me the most ridiculous question I've ever heard. He said, "ANT, how much fat do you want me to take?" I said, take *all* the fat.

I want to walk into a room with Lindsay Lohan and have people say, "Who's that fat bitch with ANT?"

I had liposuction seven times. They don't tell you that surrounding fat cells will grow back. I started getting a bunch of fat cells on my back—because if you don't change the behavior, the behavior doesn't change. I'm no different, I'm not special or unique, I just did not want to do the diet and exercise thing. I did not want to go to a gym. I felt very uncomfortable, with low self-esteem, and a gym is the last place for someone who eats their feelings. It was not a good, safe place for me.

After liposuction, I did CoolSculpting. That worked for about a hot minute.

After CoolSculpting, I went on a TV show called *The Doctors* where they got me a trainer, car rides to the gym, a free private gym membership, and delicious chef-prepared meals. I lost weight doing that show.

However, if the behavior doesn't change, the behavior doesn't change. I gained all that weight back plus more weight.

I had stomach surgery. Desperate to lose weight, I had the gastric sleeve. I lost a lot of weight, but if the behavior doesn't change, it all comes back. So I stretched my stomach out.

Brian: I know so many people who have successfully beat gastric bypass surgery.

ANT: I beat it.

Then I read about a brand-new drug out called Wegovy. People have lost up to 18 percent of their body weight using this drug.[112] On this drug I dropped from 218 to 149, no diet and no exercise. I also do a support group where they're teaching me about changing my thoughts around food. I don't eat because I'm hungry. I eat because I'm feeling something.

Brian: Like I said, I never knew you to be heavy, but apparently you were yo-yoing throughout your life.

ANT: When I'm really heavy, you don't ever see me in public.

You know, I've done crystal meth to lose weight. You lose a lot of weight really fast and you have an incredible urge to vacuum the ceiling. That wasn't the only reason I did meth, but a big reason

112 I am sure there are studies that support this statement or something similar, but this is ANT's recollection as discussed in the interview.

was weight. Our society puts so much pressure on you. Especially if you're in the public eye, it really puts a lot of pressure on you to look a certain way, even comedians.

Brian: When I first started comedy, I loved the fact that you could be of any size and be a comedian, which is technically true. But if you want to have a career or be successful, you have to look a certain way.

ANT: I think that's true for the most part, depending on what you do. You know, Ralphie May and I were very good friends, God rest his soul. Ralphie went on an audition and I helped him with the audition material. He was going in to audition for a role to play the fat guy, and the feedback came back and he didn't book the job: he was too fat to play the fat guy.

Brian: I'm glad you brought up Ralphie May, I was just thinking of him. He often said that if you are going to be overweight in comedy, you have to be ten times as funny to compensate. Of course, he was extremely funny. There are those breakout performers, but they are the exceptions to the rule.

Other than helping your public career, how does being thinner benefit you?

ANT: I want to lie to you and say it solved all my problems, but it didn't solve any problem. I wear smaller sizes and I could take my shirt off at the beach now as opposed to wearing a T-shirt in a public pool. But if you don't change your thinking and you're plagued by the same demons, being thin isn't going to change anything. When I look in the mirror, there I am.

Brian: How do you go about changing some of that internal stuff?

ANT: I'm in recovery. I'm in an eating program. The program of recovery that tells me that my thoughts are not my friend. Like, I want to beat myself up all the time. I'm at 149 right now and my head says not thin enough. When is it going to be thin enough? I don't have to listen to that. Now I can say, you know, I'm happy where I'm at right now. I'm also happy now when I'm overweight, and now I'm losing weight for different reasons than I did before. Before, I lost weight because of entertainment. VH-1 and MTV said you have to be a certain way. They had meetings about this stuff when I was hosting *Celebrity Fit Club*. They were like, you can't be fatter than the celebrity contestants.

I think now I'm more comfortable in my own skin, and that means fat or thin.

Brian: How has losing weight affected your sex life?

ANT: The quality of cock that I get has gotten larger and more plentiful. I'm kidding . . . sort of.

Brian: Nice!

ANT: I have gray hair, a gray beard, and a six-pack again. The age I'm attracting is as if I were a billionaire. I've got twenty-five and thirty-year-old men that are after me. I always say being fat and gay is like being in Frodo's ring of invisibility. Nobody fucking sees you. You lose weight and all of a sudden you're rich and famous. The world has become my oyster, Dr. Brian.

Brian: I love that. Sex and body weight are intricately linked. When I was heavier, there were times when sex seemed less appealing to me than eating a pizza. As I lose weight, my sex drive is coming back and it's much more of a motivator. Is this something you've experienced?

ANT: I'm just saying this—for every ten pounds I've lost, I masturbate ten extra times a week. I hope I don't develop a sex addiction after this. Although if I had to pick an addiction, I would take a sex addiction.

A Few Words About Medication

ANT has lost a lot of weight while taking the prescription medication Wegovy, and I have a few other friends who have also lost or are losing weight on that drug.

The first time I hit three hundred pounds, I found a clinic that prescribed Phentermine. Phentermine is an appetite suppressant that has been available in the United States since the 1960s and seemed to have a brief surge in popularity in the nineties, which coincidentally is about the time my weight hit that of a newborn elephant. It worked wonderfully for me, and I found it helped control my appetite so well that I was able to keep my calories down to under six hundred a day. This was not what the clinic had recommended, but apparently I was in a hurry.

Around six months later, I was a whole eighty pounds slimmer and at my lowest adult weight. But by the following year, I gained most of it back. And then some more. And even more after that.

I think you know how the story goes from there. The medication worked great, but the problem was that I hadn't made any lasting changes to my behavior. As soon as I went off the drug, my old habits kicked in and I just fell back into my tendency to pack on the pounds.

There are many ways to lose weight, including appetite suppressants and more severe interventions, but as ANT mentioned, "If the behavior doesn't change, it all comes back." I am sure that his weight loss was facilitated by his medication, but his continued success involves the support group he joined and the work he has done to actively change his thoughts and behavior.

Nashville Hot Chicken Restaurateur Austin Smith Lost Over One Hundred Pounds and Still Eats His Own Food

I may be writing this in Canada, but I am definitely an American. One of the awesome things about touring so much for so long was that I got to have all sorts of experiences in this wonderful, great big country of ours. I can't remember how I first learned about Nashville hot chicken, but I do know that it was before it became widespread. This was back when there were only a few spots in Tennessee serving up this deliciously painful dish. If you don't know, hot chicken started as a plate of revenge. As the story goes, Thornton Prince was a well-known ladies' man, and after a night of suspected infidelity he came home to a highly peppered plate of fried chicken. To his wife's surprise, he loved it so much, he started sharing the recipe, and years later his great-niece opened Prince's Hot Chicken Shack in Nashville. I found the story intriguing and the next time I found myself in Nashville, I had to visit Prince's. Like a lot of people, I was immediately hooked with the first bite. I made a point to try the hot chicken at all the major players in Nashville and whenever I stumbled onto it on the road. Now it seems every restaurant has some variation of Nashville hot chicken on their menu. There is even a hot chicken joint a few blocks away from me in Montreal, which I have yet to try.[113]

As I've discussed, there were a few years where I sought out interesting, and sometimes overwhelmingly big, Bloody Marys while on the road. This is what first brought Sarah and me into a newer hot chicken establishment with a great name: Party Fowl. I had seen pictures of their famous "Brunch for Two," a massive fifty-five-ounce Bloody Mary garnished with, among other things, two hot chicken-style fried Cornish game hens and two whole Scotch eggs. At the time, they were only serving four per day on weekends, but I called in advance, and given my ties in the Bloody

---

113 This is not exactly a book of weight loss advice, but even if it were, I probably shouldn't need to tell people to cut back on fried foods.

Mary community (yes, that is a thing), they reserved one for me. It was incredible and every bit worth the hype. We took notes and shot photos and then proceeded to tackle that massive drink.

As luck would have it, Austin Smith, the owner of Party Fowl, was there and we had the idea to ask him for an impromptu interview. He was extremely nice and eager to talk, so we shot one of our earliest videos (which is not very good quality, but a lot of fun). He later told us that was his first video interview. He would go on to be interviewed widely, appear on the Food Network, and even film a TV show with Shaquille O'Neal.

Over the years, Party Fowl has done really well, and Austin has opened several other locations, including one in Florida. While passing through Nashville recently, Sarah and I reached out to see if we could film another, significantly improved video, and he once again was nice enough to make time for us. After a great talk about chicken, I noticed that Austin was not the same man we first met.

Brian: You are in the restaurant business, enjoying significant success, and although everything on your menu is delicious, you're not exactly serving up health food. Fried chicken and boozy slushies aren't really on the diet for people trying to lose weight. And yet in the time since we last saw you, you've been able to slim down despite being surrounded by some of the tastiest calories in Nashville. How did you manage that?

Austin: I am proud to talk about that. About a year ago I was at 366 pounds, and I would get winded walking up my own stairs. I play softball and I tore my calf muscles three years in a row running bases, just because my body was too big and was not keeping up. I was completely out of shape and was worried that I wasn't going to live long enough to see my kids grow up, honestly. And I've got Party Fowl here and a huge family that I'm responsible to here as well.

When the pandemic hit, I said, I've never had this much time, because we were so slow. And I said, I'm gonna do it right now. I'm gonna get with a trainer and I'm gonna change everything. I stopped drinking for eight months to give it a jump-start and started tracking macros.[114] I started at four days a week lifting for an hour, doing my high-intensity training, and would then do forty minutes of cardio. As I started to see the results and I started to get everything kind of curtailed and get into a rhythm, I was like, OK, Coach, I want to add a fifth day. And then I started doing sixty minutes of cardio per day.

My first goal was to get sixty-seven pounds down and be under three hundred pounds for the first time in ten years. I got within three pounds the day before New Year's Eve, so I fasted. I'll never forget, it was 7 p.m. on New Year's Eve and I stepped on the scale. I was 298.9 and, man, I teared up. I was screaming. I called my Chinese restaurant for some Chinese food. I ate those Christmas cookies my mom had stashed away from me. I drank some red wine. I had some bourbon. I was like, give me all of the things.

So I had them all after I hit the goal, took the pictures, and made the post on social media. The next day I was back on the ground. I told my trainer I got it out of my system. I'm ready to go for the next goal. The next one was to lose a hundred pounds in

---

114 Macronutrients are those that provide us with energy: carbohydrates, proteins, and fats.

the first year. By July 13, I had hit ninety-seven pounds, but like he said, I also put on about twenty-five pounds of muscle. So I think we did good there.

For the next goal I was turning forty on March 10 and I wanted to be under 20 percent body fat, better than when I was in college. So yeah, I'm happy to talk about it. It's a kick in the ass. It is not every day you wake up and you're in that zone; you have to put yourself there.

Brian: As you know, I've had my own weight loss journey and lost about a hundred pounds. But I also don't own a fried chicken restaurant.

Austin: With a bar!

Brian: How do you manage that and still keep on track to meet your personal goals?

Austin: So our smoked beer butt chicken is phenomenal. It's sacrilegious, but I actually pull the skin off because there's too much fat in the skin, but I eat our smoked beer butt chicken a lot. I also eat the brick-tattooed chicken, which has sage and goat cheese under the skin (goat cheese is lower in fat than most cheeses), and it is delicious. I eat that dish with sautéed spinach, potatoes, bell peppers, and onions. I do the tacos grilled: two corn tortillas and a grilled tender. I've found my ways around, still getting to have my flavors and eat what I like, but doing it in a way that fits my numbers.

The biggest trick is that every vendor comes in here to pour bourbon in my glass and beer in my cup. They're like, "Hey, do you wanna try?" and I'm like, yeah . . . no. It's the worst thing ever, because I love my libations. I love little beverages. That one I have to watch, because if the liver's busy taking care of your booze it's not processing the food, and you gain everything. It sucks.

It's been a battle, but I've learned so much about me and I've learned so much about my body and I've seen the changes. I know the smallest little thing can make a change in that day, and it changes how you think. I still eat Party Fowl all the time. Every once in a while, I sneak a little hot chicken. You can get the grilled chicken dipped in that flavor.

Brian: I did get the Party Fowl grilled chicken the other night. It was delicious.

Sometimes It's Really Good to Talk to Others

The struggle for weight loss is real, and it's something I wrestle with every day. Every moment of my life I am faced with opportunities to sustain my excess body weight or attempt to whittle it down a notch. Each time I reach for food, I am deciding to either consume enough calories to keep up my already top-heavy WHR and way-too-high BMI or try to come in at a deficit and force my body to use some of the fuel it has stored away for a rainy day. Each moment I choose between calorie-burning physical activity and less calorie burning sitting on the couch. Sometimes the decisions are conscious ones, but most of the time they are made by unconscious areas in my brain. It would seem that my brain really likes sitting on the couch and occasionally getting up to browse for snacks despite my conscious desire to live healthier. My brain is a butthead.

When we are struggling, it is nice to know that we are not alone. Maybe that is the real reason I am writing this book. Perhaps by reading it, you may relate to what I have been going through, recognize some behaviors in yourself, or take comfort in knowing that you are not alone in this. Weight loss is difficult, and even though we all may know how to do it, actually doing it is the root of the battle. I found it helpful to chat with a handful of formerly heavier men and women about their struggles. It inspired and motivated me to keep on going, but also it was really good to hear from so many people dealing with the same types of issues that I am. Also it was great to catch up with some old friends, some of whom I hadn't spoken to in years and were hundreds of miles away. Sarah can attest to this, but I came away from each interview feeling positive and with a renewed appreciation for my ultimate goal. I should sit out of comedy festivals more often—this turned out to be a much better use of my time. It is really good to talk to others.

Such is the basis for group therapy and programs like Weight Watchers and Overeaters Anonymous, or any support group that meets for any purpose. When I was younger, I had workout buddies. We would regularly go to the gym together and support each other's journey, offering encouragement and accountability.

I've tried working out on my own many times, and that lasted about as long as this sentence. When I am on the road, every hotel I stay at has a small gym. Some of them are actually quite nice, and yet I can probably count on one hand the number of times I have tried to get a workout in. I'll be the first to admit that I lack discipline, because duh, that's exactly what I'm describing, but I also overwhelmingly prefer the company of other people to running on a treadmill while listening to my own thoughts. For an extrovert like me, other people make working out enjoyable. The same is true of eating and dieting. I love eating with other people. I am a social eater, but I diet alone. If I could somehow manage my consumption in the company of other people, with each of us cheering each other on and helping maintain focus, that would be rad. People don't get together to not eat. Then again, maybe they do and call it a support group.

Other people are incredibly helpful. I know a lot of people who use social media to connect with others with similar goals, checking in with each other and providing accountability. Among those I interviewed, Mark Schiff has a group he regularly checks in with, including Steve Mittleman. ANT also joined a support group. Trevin Verduzco found a clinic full of people and resources. Mark Evans began intermittent fasting with his wife. Jennifer Anderson had her weight loss tracked in front of a national TV audience. Hot chicken magnate Austin Smith hired a really good personal trainer.

I've never joined a weight loss group, but I do have Sarah and Alyssa. Sarah is amazing and supportive, and often diets with me, but she eats with me too. Alyssa helps keep me active, and her presence is a constant reminder of why I want to get healthier, but she's a kid and I don't want her to not have ice cream because her daddy is too fat. If we are out and one of us has an impulse, it isn't too hard to fall off the wagon. Those seat belts are crap. Who designed that wagon anyway?

I enjoyed talking to each of the people I interviewed, and each gave me some insight into myself.

Unlike Mark Schiff and Jonelle Larouche, I wasn't much of a drinker. I know I drank a lot of Bloody Marys in my travels, but I never developed a love for alcohol. I didn't even have a taste for it until I was living in New Orleans for graduate school. I remember one night early in my first year, a bunch of us went out for drinks at a bar just outside the French Quarter. One of my new friends was from Wisconsin, a state that knows a lot about drinking,[115] and when he noticed I was nursing a soda water, he asked me why I didn't have something harder. At parties in college, I tried whatever was available, and the taste of beer or liquor never really appealed to me. I told him I was more of a coffee drinker, and he said, "I've got the perfect beer for you," and he ordered me a stout. Boy, did he nail it. From the first sip, I was excited by this new experience and drank it down quickly. I ordered another, and another. To this day, I think I had never had good beer until that night in New Orleans. Eventually, I can say that I liked the taste of beer and other alcohol. In fact, I love beer. Once I learned about different styles and flavors, a whole new world of liquid calories opened up to my taste buds, but I still never became much of a drinker. Mainly because I didn't like being drunk. I didn't drink, I didn't

115 I would later discover that Wisconsin is also pretty serious about its Bloody Marys.

do drugs. My only consistent vice was food, and it became such a big part of my life that eating was almost all I could do to have fun.

A few of the people I interviewed were highly active people who for various reasons saw a significant reduction in their physical activity but continued to eat like Olympians. Mark Evans and my former roommate Dave DeLuca were extremely active people who gained weight because of a change in their circumstances. Each of them was able to lose about one hundred pounds by getting his behavior under control. Both were athletes who were used to disciplined behavior and healthy practices; they just needed to update their eating habits. And jump rope . . . Dave jumped a lot of rope.

One of my few regrets in life is that I've never gotten into sports. When I was a kid, my parents signed me up for sports like T-ball, but for some reason I could never get interested in them. I later learned that, like my friend Kieran Atkins, I had a case of ADHD, and perhaps that was part of it. Standing in the outfield waiting on some other kid to smack a ball off a tee in the hopes that it might come in my general direction was way too understimulating to hold my attention, and whenever a ball did pop my way, my mind was elsewhere. I never got good enough to enjoy sports, and not enjoying sports led to not being good at sports, which in turn led to being the weak link in team sports, and I hated letting people down, which further pushed me away from an interest in sports.

I wasn't an athlete, but unfortunately, I still ate like one.

In my freshman year of high school, I had some friends sign up for wrestling, and they convinced me to sign up as well. It was grueling, intense physical activity, and I loved it. Looking back,

I realize that the immediacy of the sport, with the one-on-one matches, kept my attention from straying. Wrestling is similar to fighting, and the brain is definitely not going to entertain distractions during a fight. I enjoyed it and I started to get into better physical shape; then halfway through the school year I moved to a school without a wrestling program. So much for that one. Toward my senior year in my new school, I started playing racquetball after school with some friends. Racquetball is another fast-paced activity, but I think the one-on-one aspect of both sports is what grabbed me. There were no teammates to disappoint. If I sucked, I was the only one who lost. Like wrestling, I really enjoyed it, and after a while I didn't suck.

I forget why we stopped playing racquetball, but we did. Maybe it was the end of the school year and we all went our separate ways, but whatever the reason, my brief enjoyment of the game was not enough to turn me into an athlete, and I went right back to doing something my brain loves even more: sitting on the couch.

I was really glad I talked to ANT about his experiences. I think every overweight person at some point considers the quick fixes out there. Dieting and exercise are so hard, and I often see ads for liposuction, CoolSculpting, and weight loss surgery and think maybe they could be my ticket to something quick and easy. The skeptic in me has always looked at these ads with a dubious yet hopeful eye. I have met others, like ANT, who overcame gastric surgery and gained back their weight, and that seemed to be such a horrible outcome. All that effort, pain, and money just to still be overweight a few years later. I have also met people who have undergone such treatments and kept the weight off. I never felt the odds of my being in that second group were in my favor.

It was great to talk to Erik Escobar. Not only has he been successful in losing his extra body weight, but he was so cheerful and happy. We reminisced about all the great food and beverages we enjoyed on the road. If he can successfully modify his behavior and leave that behind, then so can I.

Reaching out to and talking with these people came at a good time for me. I had lost a few of my pre-Montreal pounds, but talking about weight loss almost every day really helped keep my goals in the top of my mind, and I stuck to my guns even more. By the end of my last interview, I had lost all but four pounds of the extra weight I brought up north.

FAT TALES

Just Call Me Papa Button

The first time Alyssa saw me perform comedy, she was about two weeks old and I was headlining a small show at a bar. A lot of our family, friends, and friends of our family came out, more than usual, and I realized they were primarily interested in meeting the new baby, which, to be fair, I don't blame them for. Alyssa started stealing the show the moment she was born, and I am OK with that.

My mom and her friends were there. Comedy shows are

generally not mom or kid friendly, but this one was exceptionally raunchy. For some reason every comedian before me chose this night to test out their new blow job jokes (all of them were just as brilliant as you can imagine). Two weeks outside the womb, and my poor little girl is hearing a bunch of comics going for shock value laughs. I was so thankful that she didn't yet understand English and considered only teaching her the Nell language for her own sanity.[116] Not that I was much better: I was still pretty close to my peak weight and making all my regular jokes about being a fat guy, sprinkled in with some tasteless jokes about being a new father. Lucky for me, I recorded it.

My set included such gems as:

"Once I got to the age of thirty, I said screw condoms. What's the worst that could happen—I'm going to die in ten years. Unfortunately, that was fifteen years ago."

"I have a daughter—thankfully, because I would make a lousy role model for a boy. There's no way that nature is going to trust me to raise a male. Look how I ended up. My son would come up to me and say, 'Daddy, Daddy, teach me how to play football,' and I'd be like, dude, you teach me. If you want to learn how to play Dungeons & Dragons or read comic books, I'm your guy. On the other hand, one day my daughter is going to come to me and say, 'Daddy, Daddy, I made some brownies. Want to try them?' Hell yeah, and you might want to make another batch."

"All the clichés are true. When she was born, I was like, the hell with everything else. My comedy has gone to shit, and clearly I gave up caring about the way I dress. I have two ways that I have

116 This audience gets a reference to the 1994 Jodie Foster movie *Nell*, right?

to try on shirts now. I try them on standing up and it might seem like it fits, but then I sit down to see if I'm going to pop a button. My kid is going to grow up calling me Papa Button."

Like I said, these were gems. Golden. In the moment it was a funny set, but looking back at it now, it seems sad. I had always done self-deprecating jokes in my act, but as my health deteriorated it came across as less funny and more of a cry for help. I really did pop a button on my shirt that night. It was accidental, but I spun it into my act. The sitting belly has a different set of rules than the standing one. Papa Button even made an appearance on network TV.

For a brief month before the pandemic canceled everything, I managed to schedule a few interviews to promote *The Art of Taking It Easy*. Most of them were pretaped segments that could be edited before airing, but one was on a live morning show. I was on tour at the time, traveling with a limited wardrobe to begin with, but I thought a nice button-down shirt under a black suit jacket would give me that "casual academic" vibe I usually go for. Also, it is pretty much my standard uniform when I am on tour.

They brought me into the studio and sat me on a couch. No makeup check, no wardrobe check, just me off the street and onto the couch. I watched the anchors do their thing and learned a little about what was going on that day. During a commercial break a producer prompted me to get ready for my interview. One of the anchors joined me on the couch, and we had a delightful discussion about my book, life on the road, and managing stress. As far as I knew, all was good.

I went back to my hotel and looked for the segment online, and it was strangely missing. The rest of the morning show was available, but when I clicked the link to view my clip, it returned an error. I emailed my contact at the station, who assured me that it should be available. I even contacted the website's help desk about the error, but nobody knew why the clip wasn't working.

Thankfully, I had a local friend who watched the interview live that morning and recorded it on her phone straight from the TV. She sent me the footage so I was able to see it, and that's when I noticed something a little off. In my seated position on the couch, the force of my belly had flared the bottom button of my shirt open for the entire duration of the interview. The camera shot me straight on, giving the audience a clear view of my navel. On live TV I was outed as an innie.

I thought it was interesting that all of the anchors were wearing suits or dresses from the ankles up, with slippers and gym shoes underneath. It made sense: they were comfortable, and the part that was in frame was camera-ready. Like how nobody wore pants for online meetings during the pandemic. Given how accustomed they were to cropping out inappropriate wardrobe elements, I was surprised nobody noticed the big, gaping hole in my abdomen caught on camera.

Later that day, I received an email from our station contact who told me the clip was now available on the website and apologized for the delay. I went to watch it again and noticed they had cropped the image a bit to hide my belly button, which must have been the source of the delay: compensating for a wardrobe malfunction. So I guess that's one more thing that Janet Jackson and I have in common.

Being overweight hasn't hurt my career in any way I'm aware

of, but I could imagine it doing so. Who wants to have the belly button man on their morning news show? I wouldn't.

I always assumed that wardrobe malfunctions were a common occurrence for fat people. They definitely were for me. I've popped buttons off shirts, snapped belts off my waist, split my pants right through the crotch, rubbed holes into the inner thigh on so many jeans and shorts, and stretched T-shirts well beyond their limits. Add these to the need to constantly replace my wardrobe every time I outgrew a size, and the fact that extra large clothing costs a little more to begin with, and covering up fat becomes really expensive. It is no wonder that as I gained more and more, I let my appearance go. I became increasingly convinced that a T-shirt under a suit jacket looked good and that jeans were appropriate for any occasion. After dropping a hundred pounds, I haven't yet significantly updated my wardrobe beyond shopping in my own closet and purchasing a new suit, but I am hoping that the days of Papa Button are behind me.

8

My Boots Were Made for Walking

There is a fable about a boiling frog that I am sure you've heard before. The basic idea is that if you put a frog into boiling water, it will immediately jump out, but if you put it in tepid water and very slowly adjust the heat, it will continue to adapt to its new condition until the water comes to a boil, and you now have a delicious snack.

Before you go try this at home, sadist, you should know that it isn't true. You'll have to kill your frogs the old-fashioned way, by shoving firecrackers in their mouths. No, don't do that either, you psycho.

The fable is often used as a metaphor for psychological adaptation. If your life circumstances were to suddenly change for the worse, you would take notice and probably be pretty angry/upset/whatever. But if they gradually deteriorate, we tend to adapt to each level of discomfort and ultimately find ourselves in a position where we ask, "How did I get here?"

I asked myself that question a few years ago, in Plattsburgh, New York, while sitting in a doctor's office at my girlfriend's request to get a prescription for compression socks. Because nobody knows fashion like doctors.

How *did* I get there? For a few years leading up to my peak weight, my legs and feet had become very swollen, so much so that I hadn't worn any of my three pairs of cowboy boots in over a year. Before that, I would wear them every day. I must have toured in them for at least five or six years. I could slip them on and off easily at airports, and they didn't require much maintenance. They were versatile for the road, looked great with jeans, and were extremely comfortable. They were such a staple that they became part of my signature look. Then, slowly, things began to change. The boots started to feel tight, but I would force them on anyway. Eventually, putting them on became harder and harder. I would strain to get them over my heels, and one day I even pulled them so hard that I snapped one of the straps. By the end of a long day of standing on my feet I was unable to get them off. Sarah volunteered to help pull them off, got one off, and then fell over backward on the second one. I started to wear other, easier-to-put-on shoes more often. I had some decent-looking casual footwear for touring, and when I was home in California, flip-flops were an easy choice for most events. I adapted. I rationalized. Besides, cowboy boots are too hot for Los Angeles weather, anyway. After a while, I started having trouble bending over and crossing my legs; you know that move that is kinda essential to putting on shoes and tying laces? No worries, laceless shoes are more practical for air travel anyway

. . . until you can't squeeze your feet into them.

In Plattsburgh, right around the point when the doctor asked me if my legs "leaked" (they can do that?), I decided prescription socks were my boiling water. When we got back to Montreal, I started working on a few things, doing what I could, when I could. When we went back to the States for our next tour, I got those boots out of our storage unit to take along as a goal. A few months later, I was able to bend more comfortably, and about six months later, I was able to put my boots on without help.

Whenever I look down at my feet now, I like to admire the veins I can see across the surface and how my tendons are visible when I flex my toes. When my feet were swollen, it was nothing but smooth skin. Feet are supposed to have character.

I don't wear my cowboy boots every day now, but each time I put them on they make me smile. I never did get those fashionable compression stockings, as sexy as they may have been.

FAT TALES

A Father and Son Thing

Having lost about one hundred pounds, I look younger than I did a few years ago. I've updated my internal self-image, but when I first started to notice the change, I would be momentarily shocked every time I caught that handsome man in the mirror starring back at me. He never broke eye contact either. What a creep.

Extra weight ages a body, not just in appearance but in condition. I had aches and pains that I assumed were the result of getting older, but as they have mostly gone away I realize they were the result of getting fatter. As both of those changes take place around the same time for most human beings, it is really hard for us to separate them until one is removed.[117]

Several of the losers I interviewed mentioned that they look and feel younger than ever before. We tend to associate youth with being thin (which, unfortunately, does not ring true for every person) and think of the weight we gain as we get older as natural. But what is natural? Certainly, gaining weight as we age is a common experience, but I am not too sure it's natural. You may recall that I have an interest in evolutionary psychology. Well, I have a hard time imagining any scenario where an increase in body fat correlated with aging would be advantageous to early human beings. The prehistoric elderly probably had to outrun enemies, bears, and other predators as much as the younger members of their tribes. If they were bouncing a bowl full of jelly from their abdomens while doing so, they were going to get eaten.

Whenever I use my bear example during a public speaking appearance about stress, people often ask me if I've heard the one about the two hikers who encountered a bear. The first says to the other, "How are we going to outrun that bear?" and the other replies, "I don't have to outrun the bear, I just have to outrun you."

---

117 Weight, that is. Until someone invents some sort of de-aging technology, the extra body weight is the only one of these variables we can manipulate.

Maybe that's the missing piece. Maybe early humans survived by sacrificing the fatter, older members of the tribe to ensure their escape. Just think of all the dad jokes (like the one I just used) they were missing out on as a result. No, I don't think weight gain is natural. I think it is common given the very unnatural lives we lead in the modern world. Human bodies were not designed to sit behind a desk all day, or behind the wheel of a car, so that we can then sit in front of a television. Hell, a lot of people believe we weren't designed to sit. What a bunch of squatters.

As I gained weight, I also grew out my hair. This wasn't related to the weight gain. I had always wanted to see what I would look like with long hair and never let it grow out when I was younger. However, it didn't help. I was in my early forties, and with my hair going gray, I figured it was my last chance. I also grew out my beard for a while, either because I was experimenting with hair or trying to save money on razors. I honestly thought it looked cool. I liked to imagine I looked a bit like Sean Connery in the opening sequence of the movie *The Rock*, but in reality, I looked more like Jerry Garcia from the Grateful Dead (and sadly, he wore it better). And old. Old as fuck.

I once met an overweight woman with a lot of tattoos who told me that she got them because she thought the tattoos helped distract people from her weight.[118] Looking back, I can see how the extra hair may have subconsciously helped me hide the extra weight, at least from myself while looking in the mirror. Overweight men sporting thick beards isn't exactly a rare

118 I have my ears pierced, and she asked me if I had them done for the same reason. It seemed odd to me at the time, the idea that a couple of tiny earrings could mask a bunch of extra fat cells, but it broke the ice.

combination, either; just check out any renaissance festival, so maybe there is something to this. But like the woman with the tattoos, I wasn't fooling anyone.

So I look younger now than I did a few years ago. I keep my hair short and my beard trimmed. Hopefully, in a few years I will look younger than I do now. I'll most likely still prefer sitting over squatting, because chairs and couches are awesome.

Talking with my former roommate Dave DeLuca reminded me of an experience we shared while looking for apartments in Los Angeles. When we decided to move together, I was on the road touring and he was still living in San Francisco, so we planned to meet up in Los Angeles for two days of solid apartment hunting. We agreed to narrow our search to West Hollywood. If you are unfamiliar with Los Angeles geography, West Hollywood exists as a city within a city. It's an enclave, completely surrounded by Los Angeles except for the border it shares with Beverly Hills, another enclave. West Hollywood has its own government and rules. It is not simply the west side of Hollywood, which is technically just a neighborhood in Los Angeles. There were plenty of reasons this was attractive to us, and deciding to narrow our search to West Hollywood meant that we wouldn't be driving all over the county to look at so-called "Hollywood-adjacent" apartments. Really, Hollywood-adjacent? Maybe if you consider thirty minutes by freeway to be adjacent.

We also narrowed our search to apartments that came with parking and a pool, all within a reasonable price range of course. We then looked at two units in buildings with pools that were so disgusting we decided to drop that criterion from the search.

As comedians who often go on tour, we couldn't rely on street parking, or we'd come home from a tour to a bunch of citations for not moving during street cleaning. After eliminating the pool requirement, we noticed an improvement in the quality of units we saw, and we finally stumbled onto an absolutely great two-bedroom right off Santa Monica Boulevard. We were both happy with the place and it was in a good location, so we decided we would make an offer. The landlord gave us some applications and then asked, "So what are you guys, like a father and son thing?"

I am only about five or six years older than Dave.

We laughed it off—well, Dave laughed more than I did—and explained that we were just a couple of comedian friends. We took the applications back to the car and I promptly decided that I didn't want to live there. Dave said, "Why? That place was great!"

"Dude, he thought I was your dad!" I said. Dave could tell I was pissed, but we agreed to keep the place in the back of our minds in case we didn't find anything else. Thankfully, we found an incredible place in an amazing location, and we had an awesome few years in West Hollywood.

As I mentioned, Dave was a relentless exerciser, and remembering how we'd been misjudged got me to attempt exercising with him when we finally did move into our place. Unfortunately, I was in a bit of pain, having not yet treated my sleep apnea, and kept falling off the exercise wagon. Dave was a supportive roommate and set a good example, but at the time I found it extremely difficult to stay motivated. I sleep better now, I can handle a lot more exercise now, and overall I think I now make a much better roommate—not that I am in the market, but you never know.

During our recent interview, Dave said, "You looked like Santa Claus and I looked like one of the elves!"

I would have accepted older brother, maybe even a young uncle, but father? Fuck that guy.

9

Sarah's Struggle

I share my life with an occupational therapist, former life coach, semiprofessional tango dancer, and active art model. I know that sounds crowded, but all of those are the same person. Her name is Sarah, and she is the most beautiful woman in the world to me. She has also gained and lost a whole lot of body weight over the course of her life. It would appear that living with me is not her only struggle. I have included a few interjections from her so far throughout this book, and I think it's time we got a little more of her story.

From my wife, Sarah Bollinger:

> I previously alluded to the fact that I too have lost weight a few times in my life. I did so through different methods and lost variable amounts of weight. However, one really significant key to my weight loss has been the strength of the "why" behind wanting to lose weight and get healthy.

Do you know your why? Does it come to you like a snap, or do you have to sit down and think a moment? When you think about it, get real with yourself. Answer honestly, and be kind to yourself as if you were advising a friend.

The first time in my life I ever struggled with weight gain was in graduate school. Like many students, I kept an erratic sleeping, eating, and studying schedule. And my occupational therapy class was encouraged to remain flexible to sudden changes in our packed semester schedule. The phrase "OTs are flexible" was uttered and repeated frequently by the instructors of our program in attempts to train us for our future fast-paced health care careers. The changes happened so often that my peers often joked that the "OTs are flexible" bit was simply to cover anything the staff needed for their own scheduling needs. We gladly and enthusiastically complied because that is what we were there for and that is what we were being trained to do. It did teach me a certain degree of resilience, to roll with the punches, and to quickly adapt to changing situations and environments, and to aid my clients in adapting too. However, it did not teach me how to take care of myself while taking care of others, or more ironically yet, while teaching others how to take care of themselves while caring for loved ones. So when I set out for my first job with my Suzie Sunshine, ready-to-serve outlook, it should come as no surprise that I had also put on some weight and needed a new suit jacket to participate in interviews, as well as new, larger-sized scrubs.

After graduate school, I was also engaged to be married.[119] Like many brides, I had an idea in my head of how I wanted my dress to look and how well I wanted it to fit. The vision I had in my head did not, however, meet the one that I saw in the mirror, or match my previous level of fitness, so I set a goal to lose some weight. Wedding planning is stressful, and taste-testing menu items including three cake flavors a week does not make weight loss any easier of a task, but I did manage to lose twenty-five pounds through exercise, a personal trainer, calorie reduction, and group meetings. I didn't feel ideal, but I did feel better and a little more confident in my wedding dress.

The second time the weight came creeping back up, I was still a young clinician. I was dedicated to my work and to my patients all day, and then would exhaustedly make the long commute home, still problem-solving and thinking about them. I would arrive home, try to take a short nap on the sofa after setting an alarm, and then muster up enough energy to hit the gym before dinner and bed. A few times I slept through my alarm, only to wake up and call my trainer to apologize. (He was annoyed but still got paid.) Then I would fall back asleep, and repeat the next day, as if it were a scene from *Groundhog Day*.

Still overweight, and all the while helping my patients to get better through several methods, which included increased activity through exercise and strengthening, I couldn't help but feel a little bit hypocritical.

---

119 To some other dude. His loss is totally my gain.

I wanted to be accountable. I wanted to be an example. I wanted to feel better and be better for both myself and my patients. This time my motivational "why" was stronger, more meaningful, and more health-based. The results too were stronger. This time my methodology included dropping the personal trainer and the 5 a.m. morning yoga classes and putting down my cell phone at night (yeah, imagine that! I actually needed the sleep more), as well as menu planning, increased protein intake, and a medical clinic with weekly check-ins. I lost fifty pounds. It wasn't easy, and I learned a few more things along the way, but my motivation was also much stronger. I had daily reminders of my goals not only in the mirror but also to make the world a better place through my work. I felt more self-assured, had more energy, and had more overall leverage to support the patients I worked with.

The third time in my life I experienced major weight gain was after dealing with a series of my own traumatic medical conditions, which included an accident and major knee injury. As anyone who has suffered any medical condition knows, these things have a tendency to snowball; the human systems are connected and affect one another. Likewise, it is rare to address one body part and arrive at a simple end of story.

The injury struck me particularly hard, as earlier in the year I had been at an all-time personal high in the level of my dance skills. I was not only a prominent member and organizer in my local tango community, but I was beginning to teach and was only two weeks away from a special invite-only international tango congress in Buenos Aires, Argentina. If you've ever watched an athlete get hurt and wondered how they can simply shake it off and continue to work through the injury, I can tell you there are many reasons: high pain tolerance, the rush of protective hormones in the moment, shock, and flat-out denial.

As someone who worked in health care, has a good understanding of the human body, and is a fairly athletic person with good body awareness, I knew exactly what had happened inside my body before the imaging and lab results came back. When I walked into the doctor's office, the eyes of his interns were as wide as an owl's, and he sort of looked down at the ground, shook his head, and started with a trailing off of "I'm so sorry, Mrs. Bollinger . . ." The tone of his voice was indicating something serious, as if he had found cancer in my knee. "I didn't believe you. We can't believe you're walking."

"Walking?" I replied. "I worked in the clinic, lifted patients, and went dancing four times this week!" Eyes practically exploded out of their heads.

And then there was surgery and the rehab, a very humbling experience indeed that not only put me in in my place but later helped me to empathize more strongly with my own clients. My physical therapist at the sports and medicine center started me out with exercises like standing on one leg for two minutes with my eyes closed while using only two fingers to balance. I laughed afterward and jokingly said, "You're going to have to give me something harder. Remember, I used to be like Ginger Rogers, all high heels and backward. I used to dance with my eyes closed all night long." I kept asking for more of a challenge. I wanted to get better. One day about a week into my rehab he snapped back at me, "You should forget about dancing ever again." I was truly shocked. Up until this point I had kept it light and relatively mild.

I can tell you that as a health-care provider, sometimes having another health-care provider as a patient can be the worst. We know too much for our own good and oftentimes still don't understand each other's specialties well. However, I loved and respected physical therapists, as they had always been my team and family. I didn't want to be one of those pain-in-the-ass type of patients who also happened to be a health-care provider. Let me tell you, though—did I ever educate him and give him a piece of my mind after that statement! The session ended with my switching to another physical therapist. Oh, and I started back on a modified dancing regimen about four weeks after that.

The rehab wasn't enough to get back to normal, though. I didn't feel like myself. I had gained a mountain of weight with the combination of decreased activity and all the therapeutic bread baking and eating I had taken up. I was also riddled with other health issues and more prominently with pain. Not only in my knee, but throughout my body where inflammation and arthritis were triggered and compounded by the increased weight. I felt overwhelmed and knew I had to do something again to lose weight. I decided to go to my doctor, who I loved because he was an osteopathic doctor, always listened, and stayed up-to-date on the latest research. When I arrived, though, the wait was unusually long, and there was a new sign on the door that stated, "Please limit your number of complaints to three." I guess the word about his listening skills got out. Unfortunately for me, my list of symptoms was long, so I chose to share which ones I thought were most pertinent. He listened but chalked it up to my injury, and I came away with little more support.

Dissatisfied and still seeking answers, I decided to get a second opinion. I found a physician who not only looked at the numbers in my lab reports and listened well but asked some pertinent questions for me to reflect upon. She implied that if I stopped and asked the right questions and really wanted to address them, I may already have some of the solution to my symptoms. For example, the pain in my right hip and shoulder could also be related to a long work commute. Might I want to consider a job closer to home? Perhaps my acne, insomnia, and reproductive issues also had similar lifestyle choice linked to them. OK, so yeah, let's address the elephant . . . or bear . . . in the room if you haven't already picked up on it (which would be natural, as I didn't realize it and I was living it): I wasn't exactly living a stress-free life.

I left that day with an appreciation of the doctor's more holistic approach and acknowledgment that there is always room for improvement in health. I realized that my many problems might require many solutions. From then on, I sought out an approach to my weight loss and health that was geared toward a broader perspective that addressed overall lifestyle, health, and wellness. My "why" for becoming healthy was much stronger than simply wanting to fit into a dress, much stronger than simply wanting to set an example for others, but was about myself: to thrive again in my dance skills and to find an optimal level of health.

FAT TALES

The Day After Thanksgiving

Before coming up to Montreal we were in Dallas, and on the day after Thanksgiving, I had an appointment at a nearby clinic to review my test results from a recent physical. At the time I was feeling fine, but it had been a few years since I'd had a checkup, and because I was fifty years old, they tested everything. Seriously, *everything*.

I brought my family with me, not because I felt I needed the support but because that's just how we do things. Plus, as Sarah is a health-care professional, I like to have her present whenever I do anything medical. I knew she would take notes, ask the right questions, and remember to follow up on anything we needed to do next. Alyssa didn't like the boring clinic, but she was well behaved for the most part.

We had only met the doctor once before, on the day of my physical about a month earlier, but he had been listed as my primary care provider the entire time we lived in Dallas. For over a year this man's name was on my insurance card, but I had never used it and had only reluctantly scheduled the physical because of Sarah. Still, he remembered us and even commented on things that would not have been recorded in our chart. He asked if I had started touring again and even remembered that Sarah is a physical therapist (she's an occupational therapist, but that was damn close). He was a nice guy, and it was a shame I waited so long to introduce myself.

I hadn't wanted to go because I knew most of my health concerns were related to my weight and that as I lost body fat, I would ultimately get healthier. Plus, nice guy or not, why should I part with my hard-earned copay money just to get an official attaboy from my doctor? Sarah convinced me to get the physical because we were going to be leaving Texas soon and I remembered what happened the last time she had me get a physical, so yeah. When Sarah says go to the doctor, you better go to the effing doctor.

Since it was the day after Thanksgiving, I was still carrying a belly full of turkey and pie, so I consciously overlooked the results on the scale. The good news started rolling in during my vitals when my blood pressure was the lowest I could remember it being. It was so low, I questioned the instrument. I doubted the person who took it. I had to reconfirm. Sarah just smiled. When the doc started going over the test results, one by one he would state that I was in the normal or healthy range for everything. Blood sugar was normal, cholesterol was low, kidneys and liver seemed to be functioning great. Even things that may not have been directly related to my weight were all coming up roses. There is something really awesome about having a medical professional go over a list and explain all the ways you are in good health. It felt amazing and was worth at least two copays. I'm not sure what's standard, but I tipped him 15 percent.

Since the birth of my daughter, I have managed to lose about one hundred pounds, as you know . . . and as we walked out to the car I looked at Sarah and Alyssa, these two women who helped me get my life on track, and all I could do was smile. We hopped into the car, and as I put on my seat belt, I told Sarah that unfortunately she may have to wait a little longer for her free condo.

The crazy thing is that I still had a lot to lose, but I had come a long way. My doctor confirmed what I had already known: that I was getting healthier. As our time in Texas was coming to an end and we were heading to Montreal and possibly another tour, I wondered how long it would take me to lose the rest of my weight.

10

Au Revoir de Montréal

Well, we have reached the end of the summer and are getting close to the end of the book. We had an absolutely awesome time reconnecting with our favorite city, seeing some old friends, and making some new ones. Being back after four years away reminded Sarah and me why we fell in love with this city in the first place, and I think it helped add a little spark to the love we feel for each other as well.

I was especially happy that Alyssa loved it. She was in a stroller the last time we were here, not even a year old, so everything was new to her. She loved the parks, exploring Old Town, the festivals (MURAL Festival was her favorite[120]), and developed an appreciation for French bread, particularly baguettes. She even asked if we could sign her up for French lessons so she could talk more

120 There was a cheese company giving out slices of pizza as a promotion, and anywhere a kid can get free pizza is naturally going to stand out in memory.

with one of our neighbors. My five-year-old literally asked to learn French! Maybe someday she can teach Sarah and me.

We are now preparing to head back to the States. We have already gotten rid of everything we can and are packing the rest in and on top of our car in the morning for the drive south. Like every other snowbird, we will be heading for the border soon. Our first stop will be in Plattsburgh, and then we are off to New York City to visit the office of my publisher before heading back on tour to Colorado, Montana, and Utah. I think it is going to be an amazing tour.

Oh, and I got rid of all of the weight I gained before we arrived. I am happy to say that I am now back down to one hundred pounds lost despite having a few plates of poutine and a little too much maple syrup. I still have more to lose, but after writing this book for the last few months and interviewing others about their journeys, I am armed with more inspiration.

Epilogue

Why has it taken me so long? One hundred pounds is a lot of weight to lose, and I am proud of myself for doing it and happy that I have made it this far. However, it has taken me over five years to get to this point, and if I am doing my math correctly, that is an average of twenty pounds a year. Only twenty? I feel like I should be able to lose twenty pounds by skipping breakfast!

Plus, I still have a way to go. A guy recently asked me, "Are you still trying to lose weight?" I answered, "Am I skinny yet?"

Each of us has our own obstacles to overcome. My obstacles include the simple fact that I have a strong attraction to food and dining experiences. I eat for many reasons that have nothing to do with hunger: I eat to be social, I eat out of boredom, and I eat for entertainment. Throughout my life, eating has so consistently been a source of positive reinforcement to my brain that I doubt I can ever forget how to find good restaurants or suppress my desire for doughnuts when triggered. I spent nearly forty-five years training my brain's unhealthy tendencies, and it could be a while before I completely overcome them. I think the same is true for a lot of us. The pursuit of better health is difficult but not impossible, and for once I have decided to put forth some serious effort. I am capable of losing my extra body weight. We all are. It might just take some time.

I also have a career that keeps me away from home, when I have a home, for months at a time, and I am largely dependent on the kitchens of professionals for sustenance. I have always observed that my behavior is easier to regulate at home. When I am stocking my own kitchen and preparing my own meals, I can and do make healthier choices for myself. I demonstrated that over the summer in Montreal, successfully losing the weight I had put on from the previous tour. Keep in mind this was weight that I had lost and gained back several times already. I am really starting to hate the yo-yo. Each three- to four-month tour seems to bring that yo-yo back up a few notches and extend my waistline a few inches.

For this reason, Sarah and I left Canada with a plan to change some of our usual touring habits. We brought along a cooler so that we could carry groceries on the road instead of eating out so much. We stocked fresh vegetables for salads, fruits for snacks, lean meats to make sandwiches for lunch, microwavable popcorn to enjoy when we settled into our hotel rooms, and bottles of unsweetened iced tea and coffee to avoid stopping at cafés. We also brought a bathroom scale to regularly check our progress.

It was an especially packed tour, with speaking gigs, comedy shows, book signings, and rare opportunities to visit with friends we hadn't seen in ages. Ultimately, touring means a lot of driving, and this tour, which was mostly across the western states, was no exception. During my daytime seminars, I functioned perfectly well on the groceries we brought, but travel between cities was tough. There were long stretches of highway where we found an apple just wasn't going to cut our need for sustenance, so I allowed myself to indulge slightly when I felt I needed more of an energy boost. And maybe I indulged a few times too many. Also at least once a week, we treated ourselves to a nice meal to reward jobs[121] well done.

Sarah was watching her calories as well, and it was helpful to do it together. Monitoring our weights with the scale was a fantastic idea. Every other day I could see if I was starting to gain and modify my behavior accordingly. I fluctuated and Sarah did too, but at the end of the first month we were both the same weight we were when we began the tour. Neither of us got closer to our long-term goals, but we were able to keep the yo-yo from bouncing back up, and I count that as a win.

I fully believe that establishing some sort of accountability can be helpful to achieve any goal. Grades in school, performance reviews in work, and deadlines imposed by publishers are all wonderful (if annoying) motivators to help achieve professional goals.

Often with personal goals there is no external authority holding us accountable. Although my family is concerned about my health, nobody is monitoring my weight loss but me. I don't have regular check-ins with anyone outside my home, and my progress (or lack of) is entirely up to me. A lot of people with my

121 On tour, Sarah works as my manager and Alyssa is homeschooled. We all work on the road.

circumstances turn to groups on the internet for accountability, but that still requires regular updates and activity.

I could use a good support group. As someone who is trained in psychology, I recognize the therapeutic value of support groups and always recommend them to others, so why not join one myself? Or maybe even start one? I was highly motivated and inspired as I was interviewing my friends who have lost weight.

It is often mentioned that although stand-up comedy is an art form for individual performers, none of us could do what we do without other comedians. Comedians often start at open mics produced by other comedians and attended by even more comedians in the audience. Eventually we develop our skills and start booking showcases with lineups of other comedians. Maybe we go on tour with a few others or get hired to host or feature for a headlining comedian. Maybe we book a gig in a club that was opened by a comedian. The point is that for years I have recognized that no comedian is an island and perhaps I should treat weight loss the same way by involving more people in the process.

On that note, I will say that there are few things that will get you back into weight loss mode like trying to write a book about losing weight. Some people comment that writing a book is hard, but so is losing weight. I figure if I can do one, why can't I do the other? According to Sarah, the hardest part of going to the gym is actually getting to the gym. As of now, I have written another book—now I just have to make sure I don't gain a bunch of weight before it is published. How is that for accountability?

The struggle is real, but we can all live healthier and better lives. I may be on the right track. I am healthier, I feel better, and I have more energy than I did five years ago. I look and feel younger. In fact, two days before turning over this manuscript to my publisher, I went to a doctor for a checkup. The doctor looked at my age and did a double take. She said that I do not look like I am fifty-one, that I look much younger than that. I think she knew that by saying so, she would be included in my new book about how to look younger by losing weight. So here it is. Also, we have a date in two months.

Good luck with your struggle.

Acknowledgments

Look, Mom, a third book!

There are hundreds of people who have helped me get to this point, and to all of them I am extremely grateful. Whether they provided support, guidance, or encouragement along the way, I appreciate how fortunate I have been to have had such good people in my life. My sincere thanks goes out to you all even if I don't mention everyone by name.

First I'd like to thank my daughter, Alyssa, who came into my life just when I needed her the most. She is a wonderful human being and I love the time I have with her. At five, she is already learning to read and I hope she someday enjoys Daddy's books from inside the covers.

Of course I would like to thank my wife, Sarah Bollinger, for her contributions to this book and just for being the awesome person she is. When I first pitched this project to my publisher, I knew that I wanted Sarah involved. Not only has Sarah helped me on a personal level with my health, but she is a gifted writer and I am extremely thankful for her input. As in life, she helps balance my silliness with a bit of pragmatism.

I would like to thank my publisher, Apollo Publishers, and specifically Julia Abramoff for giving me this opportunity. Julia has now worked with me on all three of my books, and has added a bit of class to them all.

I would like to thank my brother, Jon, and my parents, Clyde and Debbie, for being so supportive over the years.

I would like to thank all of the friends and comedians who I interviewed for inspiration in this book. I thoroughly enjoyed our discussions and feel that each of the interviews adds valuable perspectives to my overall narrative. Please be sure and check out their work as well.

In order of appearance:

Andrew Ginsburg, www.andrewginsburg.com

Suzi Gerber, author of *Plant-Based Gourmet*

Thomas Nicolai, www.thomas-nicolai.de

Mark Schiff, www.markschiff.com

Steve Mittleman, www.twitter.com/stevemittleman

AC Valiante, www.instagram.com/ac_valiantecomedy

Jonelle Larouche, www.jonellelarouche.com

Trevin Verduzco, www.instagram.com/trevinverduzco1

Mark Evans, www.southernnotstupid.com

Kieran Atkins, www.londonweighttraining.co.uk

Jennifer Anderson, podcast "Bacon with Mike and Jenn" on Spotify

Erik Escobar, www.instagram.com/erikescobar

Dave DeLuca, www.daveishere.com